Lunchtime Walks

Akuzike Nkhalamba

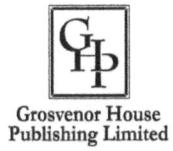

Grosvenor House
Publishing Limited

All rights reserved
Copyright © Akuzike Nkhalamba, 2025

The right of Akuzike Nkhalamba to be identified as the author of
this work has been asserted in accordance with Section 78
of the Copyright, Designs and Patents Act 1988

The book cover is copyright to Akuzike Nkhalamba

This book is published by
Grosvenor House Publishing Ltd
Link House
140 The Broadway, Tolworth, Surrey, KT6 7HT.
www.grosvenorhousepublishing.co.uk

This book is sold subject to the conditions that it shall not, by way of
trade or otherwise, be lent, resold, hired out or otherwise circulated
without the author's or publisher's prior consent in any form of
binding or cover other than that in which it is published and
without a similar condition including this condition being
imposed on the subsequent purchaser.

A CIP record for this book
is available from the British Library

Paperback ISBN 978-1-83615-499-0

INTRODUCTION TO LUNCHTIME WALKS

This book is inspired by lunchtime walks with my sister during lockdown. The genre of this book is therefore a lifestyle self-help book which includes the lessons I have learnt throughout my life and the growth that I have experienced through these lessons. The subject matter of this book is my life journey to date as a black immigrant woman living in the UK. In this book, I will go through a range of topics which include my relationships, health (both mental and physical), spirituality, finances and career journey.

I will go through each topic in the form of a business lifecycle,[16] explaining how each cycle has had an impact on my life. The cycles will include:

1. Existence – in this cycle I will go through each part of my life from my childhood (where it all started).
2. Survival – in this cycle I will go through how I went into survival mode in each area of my life.
3. Success – in this cycle I will go through how I started seeking tools to help me manage each area of my life better.

4. Take-off – in this cycle I will go through how I started using tools to manage each area of my life better.
5. Resource maturity – in this cycle I will go through how I started being consistent with each tool to ensure longevity.

The structure of this book will go through each topic relating it to each phase of the business life cycle, therefore:

Chapter 1 – Relationships – Existence	1
Chapter 2 – Relationships – Survival	5
Chapter 3 – Relationships – Success	9
Chapter 4 – Relationships – Take Off and Resource Maturity	14
Chapter 5 – Career – Existence	18
Chapter 6 – Career – Survival	23
Chapter 7 – Career – Success	28
Chapter 8 – Career – Take Off and Resource Maturity	32
Chapter 9 – Spirituality – Existence	35
Chapter 10 – Spirituality – Survival and Success	38
Chapter 11 – Spirituality – Take Off and Resource Maturity	44
Chapter 12 – Health – Existence	48
Chapter 13 – Health – Survival and Success	52

Chapter 14 – Health – Take Off and Resource Maturity	55
Chapter 15 – Finances – Existence and Survival	58
Chapter 16 – Finances – Success	62
Chapter 17 – Finances – Take Off and Resource Maturity	66

I will also take you through various topics that have spoken volumes to me over the years. These topics are: Vulnerability, The Power of Manifestation, Staying Connected, The Value of Community, Isolation, Imposter Syndrome, Single Season, Preparing for Marriage, Self-Care Vs. Soul Care, Boundaries and Discipline & Consistency.

Chapter 18 – Vulnerability	69
Chapter 19 – The Power of Manifestation	74
Chapter 20 – Staying Connected	78
Chapter 21 – The Value of Community	82
Chapter 22 – Isolation	86
Chapter 23 – Imposter Syndrome	89
Chapter 24 – Single Season	93
Chapter 25 – Preparing for Marriage	95
Chapter 26 – Self-Care Vs. Soul Care	97
Chapter 27 – Boundaries	99
Chapter 28 – Self-Discipline & Consistency	101

ABOUT ME

Hi, my name is Aku. I was born in a small town in Malawi called Thyolo in the year 1992. At the age of four, my parents decided to uproot the family to the UK. Whilst in the UK, my father studied for his master's and then later on his PhD at the University of Reading.

As a young child, I saw my parents work extremely hard whilst juggling work, studies and raising four children (my two older sisters, my younger brother and I). Regardless of their busy schedules, my parents always ensured that we were well dressed, well fed and most importantly had some family time. I remember the joyous family car trips in which we would listen to my father's CDs, memorising all the songs. This is where my love for music came from. We also took family day trips to London. My mother would make an assortment of food which we would pack to take on the trips.

Once my father graduated from his PhD in the year 2000, my parents decided to move the family back to Africa. We first landed in Malawi and stayed with relatives. We then moved to Mozambique where my father had found a job. It was difficult finding English-speaking schools in Mozambique, primarily for my eldest sister who was in secondary school. My father's friend had told him about a boarding school in Swaziland which was a few hours' drive from Mozambique. When asked whether my other sister and I wanted to join our eldest sister at boarding school, we jumped at the opportunity, therefore leaving my younger brother in Mozambique with my parents as he was not old enough. Boarding school was an extremely tough transition from what I was used to. It was the first time I witnessed teachers hitting students for bad behaviour or even the slightest of mistakes. This made me work extremely hard to ensure I did not have to endure this punishment. It made me take education very seriously and made me want to aim for only positions one, two or three in my class (position one = top achiever in the whole class followed by position two and three).

We then moved to South Africa in 2001 and my mother got a teaching job at the school we were enrolled in. Alongside this, my parents opened a grocery store as their first business venture. With my mother being a teacher at the school, my father being a PhD-holder and having experienced the boarding school in Swaziland, I was keen to continue with my hard work at school. I aimed to achieve either position numbers one, two or three in my class. I managed this well and would compete with the top three achievers in the whole class with the aim of beating them to position number one.

In the year 2003, my parents decided to move the family back to the UK after some challenges faced in South Africa. It was a hard transition coming back to the UK and trying to fit. It made me feel very insecure to the point that I shut down and became extremely shy. Although I managed to make friends and remain a high achiever in my secondary school years, I was in my shell.

Going to university after getting in through the clearing process (more explained on this journey in the chapters of this book), helped me to come out of my shell and I began to see my personality shine through. After university, my life as an adult started. This transition was challenging (explained more in the chapters of this book). I had to find ways to navigate through adulthood in the best way I could. There have been ups and downs, but I am truly grateful to God for the journey. He has taken me on and is still taking me on as I continue to discover myself. I hope you enjoy the chapters of this book as I share my journey with you.

INTRODUCTION

I have definitely evolved from the young, insecure, shy girl who did not want to put myself out there (not to say I don't have my days but I have developed a Self-Care Toolkit (mentioned in a section of this book) to pick me up when I am having 'one of those days'). Now, I am a woman, independent and open enough to share my experiences – the lessons I have learnt, the challenges I have faced and the knowledge I have gained. We sometimes go through life keeping our experiences to ourselves but through sharing our experiences, I have seen that we often share things in common. We listen to others and can relate to their story, or we listen and offer support in various ways. This gives me great joy as it shows a sense of togetherness and that we do not have to walk this journey of life alone. I have written this book because I often felt that I was going through my experiences of life alone, but the more I have shared and the more I have seen others share I have seen that others have gone through and are going through similar situations. My hope is for this book to offer encouragement to anyone reading this through each element and phase of their life and to stay reminded that there is always hope. Romans 12:12 reads 'Rejoice in hope, be patient in tribulation, be constant in prayer'. The journey of life can take us in so many directions and there is power in finding the things that keep us grounded which I will go through during this book.

As mentioned at the start, this book is inspired by lunchtime walks with my sister during lockdown. We secured our first home in December 2019 after saving up tirelessly whilst living with our parents. It was a long journey that took a lot of hard work but finally, at the age of 27, I was officially a homeowner! We were so thrilled and proud of ourselves! There were some minor improvements that we wanted to make before fully living in the house including changing the carpets, painting the whole house and making it feel like home. We immediately got to work so that, by the end of February 2020, we had completed these first steps and had bought some furniture – beds being on the top of the list. We were in the process of looking for more furniture and decorating when suddenly we were hit by the news of the Covid-19 pandemic and lockdown. Luckily, my sister and I had done enough to move into the house!

During the early stages of lockdown, my sister and I spent time watching our favourite TV shows, cooking lovely meals and most importantly getting out there and getting some fresh air. We were both working from home so going for walks was very key during lockdown to ensure we remained sane. It was great exploring our neighbourhood, having lovely walks in the park and just talking about life. We would often get into deep conversation about our careers, relationships, our health (both mental and physical) and spirituality. These discussions have formed the chapters that you are about to read from my perspective and my own personal journey.

And what a journey it is... life! The countdown to my 30s has definitely taught me a lot of valuable lessons... it has been a journey and the journey continues. We often ask ourselves what we would say to our younger selves today. There is so much I would say to that young little girl as she now continues to discover herself as a woman each day. Dear younger self:

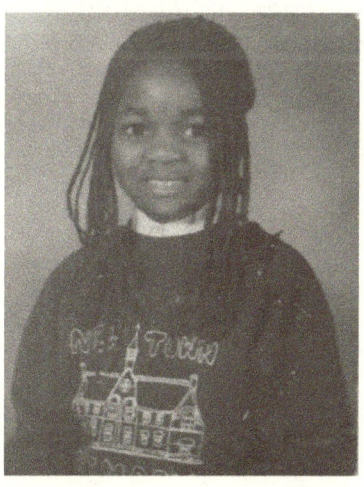

James 1:2-4 reads 'Consider it a great joy, my brothers, whenever you experience various trials, knowing that the testing of your faith produces endurance. But endurance must do its complete work, so that you may be mature and complete, lacking nothing'.

Through this journey of life, God has guided me through every season. He is continuing to guide my steps to this very day. Life can test us in various ways. Someone's test may look different to another person's test depending on the path that has been set ahead of them. The tests can either make us or break us; however, I believe that having faith no matter what life throws at us is essential to getting us through whatever season we are going through. It is not always easy and definitely tough at times, but I have found that having faith over fear through the ups and downs of life is definitely worth it. I will elaborate more on this during the Spirituality chapters of this book.

RELATIONSHIPS – EXISTENCE

Relationships, relationships... what can I say? There are so many dynamics to relationships, where to start! I have always been the kind of person who treasures relationships, regardless of whether they are familial, platonic or romantic.

Growing up, I was definitely a people pleaser. I was extremely sensitive to the moods of others, keenly observing expressions and behaviours and going out of my way to serve, to please and to avoid conflict – even at my expense.

This showed up in all forms of relationships. As a child, I would always aim to please my parents. I wanted to be the model child who would work hard at school so that I could come home with good grades and make them proud. I would also come home and, without even being asked, do all my chores. I was so eager to please!

I grew up with my three siblings – two older sisters and a younger brother. As the youngest girl in the family, culturally, I was the one who would get sent most to do certain chores around the house. I also took it upon myself to go above and beyond to show that I was fulfilling my 'duties'.

I did not mind having this role within the family as it worked well – I just got on with it and did what I was 'supposed' to do without ever questioning anything. I would listen obediently to my older sisters and parents as, culturally, to do otherwise would be considered disrespectful.

As I grew older and started developing romantic and platonic relationships, I realised how the same patterns I had developed in my family relationships were showing up.

In friendships, I would do the same and go above and beyond to make sure I was being the best friend I could be and did not question much. I always wanted to keep the peace. Confrontation did not exist in my world. I thought of confrontation as something that would ruin my relationships.

The same behaviours showed up in romantic relationships in which I would want to please the person I was with by not confronting some of the things I was unhappy with. In my early 20s I was set on finding the man that I would spend the rest of my life with – I was determined to meet my target of matrimony by the age of 25! This came from having conversations with friends from the age of 15 in which I was so sure that by the age of 25 I would have my dream job, husband and kids (25 just seemed like that 'I've got it together kinda age'). I had always viewed this as the standard route for my life and little did I know that there were spanners in the works and that no matter how meticulously I planned it all out in my head, life has so many outcomes. I would get into relationships on the basis that we liked each other and I was somehow sure that somewhere along the line the marriage and the kids would fall into place as it is 'supposed' to. I was unclear about the rest of the things that I wanted in the relationship and thought that the love, kids and house would satisfy all. Being unclear made me question certain things when I was in a relationship such as my values, beliefs and how the person I was with treated me – are they respectful? Do they value my opinions? Are they supportive? Are they open with me? Do they have the capacity to lead in a diligent manner? I did not have many deal breakers in my early 20s which meant I let things slide and disregarded some of my values and beliefs.

This is an introduction to how my view of all relationships started. I had to decide whether this approach to relationships was going to continue or change. In life, when we are uncertain about how to change situations for our own good, we often go into survival mode to keep things moving without realising the stressful impact this is having on us.

Colossians 3:23 reads 'Whatever you do, work at it with all your heart, as working for the Lord, not human masters'. This verse has so much meaning and at this point in my life I was unaware of the value this verse had. The start of my relationships was definitely a sign that I was putting all my strength in pleasing those in my life. It can be hard to break away from habits that have been formed from childhood. These habits can follow us into adulthood if we do not take the time and opportunity to fully analyse the reasons for our behaviours. In this instance, the behaviour for me was having the constant need to please others.

In the next chapter, 'Relationships – Survival', I will take you through the development of my relationships, detailing the ways in which I literally went into 'survival mode' and the impact this had on me and those close to me.

RELATIONSHIPS – SURVIVAL

In the last chapter, 'Relationships – Existence', I wrote about how I went into survival mode to keep things moving in my relationships. Survival mode meant that I continued to avoid confrontation at all costs in all forms of my relationships. I did not have boundaries and would agree to do things I was not 100% happy with. If I was asked to do something that I did not have the capacity to do, my immediate response would often be 'yes' whilst sometimes internally complaining to myself, asking myself why I had agreed to something when I had a million other things to do?

It was in my mid-20s that I began to truly see the effect this was having on me. Going above and beyond in my relationships was becoming exhausting. In some relationships I could see myself constantly giving without receiving. Regardless of this, I continued to do it. I thought that if I stopped giving so much of myself to people, then I would lose that bond and relationship with them – this scared me. I thought that going above and beyond showed people how much I truly cared about them. If asked by a family member, friend or significant other to do something at short notice, I was often there ready with the response 'yes', even though it meant juggling a few other things that I had already planned.

I later felt like I was losing control of my own life and plans by being at the beck and call of others. I did not know how to express myself without 'hurting anyone's feelings'. Not knowing how to express myself left me feeling stuck in some relationships. In my familial relationships I felt stuck because of the guilt of saying 'no' to a family member, feeling the need to be there whenever they wanted me to be. Anything less was not good enough. I had also become so accustomed to pleasing people that the word 'no' did not come naturally. This created a barrier as I often felt I could not freely communicate about certain things for fear of upsetting or disappointing a family member. This was a similar thing in some of my friendships where I thought being a good friend meant not disappointing your friends and again saying 'yes' to things even though I did not have the capacity to do them.

In my romantic relationships I also felt stuck because I was so keen on making the relationship work that I would ignore red flags. As mentioned in my earlier chapter, there are things that I started to question in certain relationships I was in. I went on dates ignoring things such as someone cutting me off mid-sentence, someone finding some of my values 'ridiculous' or someone failing to communicate with me, leaving me guessing their thoughts and feelings. I figured, *if they like me then what does it matter?* Well, all I can tell you now is that it matters a whole lot! I would often give someone multiple chances to show me that the red flags I was getting from them were not part of their true character, often being misled. I would also make excuses for them, forming reasons in my mind for their actions and giving them the benefit of doubt. I would then later realise that I had wasted time investing myself into something that was not going to give me what I needed or wanted out of a romantic relationship. I also found that certain people I would date would take advantage of my people pleasing ways and willingness to make the relationship work.

I persisted with my people pleasing tendencies to keep the peace in various relationships. As mentioned before, I was exhausted and not sure what I needed to do to get myself out of the rut I was in. Being in survival mode was an awful feeling!

Initially, I was not aware that I was in survival mode, I was just getting on with the demands of the world and others – 'fulfilling my duties'. One day during lockdown when everything remained still and silent, surrounded by four walls, I sat there and tears from nowhere began to fall. I sat there crying for a while not being able to pinpoint the problem. After all the discussions I had had with my sister during our walks, I could not bring myself to tell her what the problem was. It was a moment of self-reflection that made me realise how exhausted I was feeling. I felt as though I had been continuously pouring into people and was not getting much back. I then finally looked at my sister and said to her, 'I feel as though I have nothing left to give.' I knew at this point that I had a lot of inner work to do in terms of my relationships.

I just wanted the numbness to disappear and I yearned to have healthy boundaries in my relationships without feeling the need to say 'yes' to everything. I have learnt that in life when we are not feeling the way we want to feel, we need to do whatever it takes to get to the bottom of that feeling. We then need to take the necessary steps to get to where we want to be by taking the chance to learn and grow. This to me is SUCCESS! That brings us into the next chapter, 'Relationships – Success'.

Isaiah 41:10 reads 'So do not fear, for I am with you; do not be dismayed, for I am your God. I will strengthen you and help you; I will uphold you with my righteous hand'. This verse speaks volumes. As mentioned above, trying to please those in my life without having any boundaries broke me to the point in which I felt empty. At this point I had not yet received the revelation that the best relationship I can ever build is with God. Through my relationship with God, I can learn to have better relationships with those in my life. I have now found that relying on God's strength is the best source for me. I have learnt that building a strong connection and relationship with God is key. Along with God's strength, talking to someone who can give sound advice is helpful too. I will go through this in the next chapter.

RELATIONSHIPS – SUCCESS

In the last chapter, I wrote about how, when we are not feeling the way we want to feel, we need to do whatever it takes to get to the bottom of that feeling. Taking these steps to me is 'success'. In the last chapter, I shared how I knew I had to find a way of getting to the bottom of my feelings and started to look into my options. At this point in time, I was 28. I decided to speak to my GP who referred me to CBT (cognitive behavioural therapy) which is a talking therapy that can help you manage your problems by changing the way you think and behave. It's most commonly used to treat anxiety and depression, but can be useful for other mental and physical health problems. More on this can be found on the NHS website.[1]

I started the CBT programme. I was given an online course to go through which I would discuss weekly with a therapist, checking in on my progress. The online courses had very useful information and the therapist I was assigned helped explain things further. At first, I found it useful as this was the first time I had sought out something that may help me understand my thoughts and feelings. However, as I continued the programme, I knew that it was not going deep enough for me and I needed more. I decided to research what else was available. I saw the value of speaking to a professional and wondered if I could find someone who would better understand my background and journey.

I went looking and found a black female therapist a few months after I turned 29. My first session was not what I expected. I was only hoping to tackle the relational issues I was experiencing in the present moment but when my therapist asked me to go through my whole journey to present, it surprised me when tears began to flow. I felt really embarrassed crying in front of a stranger, something I rarely did. Normally I would hold it in thinking that crying in front of strangers would make me look weak exposing my weaknesses to them. As I cried, I kept apologising to my therapist, who was extremely understanding and encouraged me to let it out. After that session, I felt like a weight had been lifted off of my shoulder and I looked forward to the next one.

During my sessions, my therapist would ask me to walk through the journey of each form of my relationships. In my familial relationships we went through how I was stuck in the position of being the sister and daughter who did not want to rock the boat but how as an adult I wanted to break away from that and be seen as the adult I am. Not knowing how to break away from that meant that if I was unhappy with something I would give family members the silent treatment hoping that they would see how angry I was, and this would somehow fix the problem. I took this same attitude into some of my friendships and romantic relationships too. I would also act in a passive aggressive manner in all forms of my relationships hoping that people would see how unhappy I was without really explaining what the problem was. If the person didn't get the signal, I would then fume internally – and to whose benefit? My therapist spoke to me about the ways in which I could communicate my thoughts and feelings – something I had never been comfortable with. However, as they say, 'to reach success, we must get out of our comfort zone' – this is true on so many levels. Talking this through with my therapist made me realise how I needed to change my approach in the way I addressed my family, friends and anyone I was in a relationship with.

I also spoke to my therapist about how I just wanted to close the door on the shy, insecure younger version of myself as I hated how limited I felt she was. My therapist made me realise how I could not shut the door on her completely. Although I could only see the limitations, my younger self was also very kind, generous and sweet and those are the things I realised I wanted to hold onto. To me, growing and evolving is about becoming better versions of ourselves, therefore working on the things that we need to do to progress but it is also holding onto things that still make us shine.

Therapy was giving me the tools that I needed to manage all forms of my relationships. I learnt that nurturing relationships does not mean saying 'yes' to everything – it means setting healthy boundaries and if those boundaries cannot be respected then there is a flaw in that relationship that needs to be addressed.

I started practising this in all my forms of relationships by making it clear how I felt and also looking out for toxic behaviours in relationships so that I can manage them better.

From this I learnt that I am only truly in control of my actions. I learnt that I can distance myself from toxic situations/people and although there will be times in which we cannot fully distance ourselves from toxic people, we can walk away from toxic situations. I have also learnt that it is possible to love toxic people from a distance, an approach that honours my needs as much as the other party's.

In my family relationships I noticed that communication had improved in a big way due to the tools I had learnt and started to use. Instead of the passive aggressive approach I would typically use, I began to really talk through situations and was amazed by how well this was received by my family. The same goes for my friendships. There are times when I sense disappointment from family or friends when I say no, but I have realised that to look after myself, I need to be realistic with what I can do and handle so that I can show up as the best version of myself in all forms of my relationships. Disappointment is a part of life and going above and beyond to avoid it is unrealistic.

I have previously mentioned conversations I had with my friends at the age of 15 stating that I would be married by 25. Having dated and not married by that age was disappointing. The questions I would get about this from friends and family served to highlight my 'failure'. I saw friends settling down and wondered, *what is wrong with me?* My healing journey was teaching me not to settle for anything less than what I deserved. Although it was tempting to ignore red flags, I knew that a relationship that did not meet my needs would leave me unfulfilled in the long run.

Therapy was helping me to put things into perspective, giving me what I needed to create healthy boundaries in my relationships and making me realise that saying 'no' was not the end of the world. It also helped me to filter out so much negativity that I was clinging onto. I started to feel as though I could breathe again. This takes us into the next chapter, 'Relationships – Take Off'. When we continue to use the tools we have gained to become a better version of ourselves, we then have to learn to become consistent. Consistency allows the tools to become a lifestyle.

Ephesians 4:29: 'Do not let any unwholesome talk come out of your mouths, but only what is helpful for building others up according to their needs, that it may benefit those who listen'. Building healthy relationships by being self-aware is so vital. It is helpful in interacting with others by ensuring that our words or actions are not harmful towards others. When I read this verse, it made me realise that as well as protecting myself from unhealthy relationships, I need to make the effort of checking myself when interacting with others by ensuring that my words and actions are not harmful towards others.

RELATIONSHIPS – TAKE OFF AND RESOURCE MATURITY

In the last chapter, I wrote about how I started using therapy as a growth tool to help me create healthy boundaries in my relationships. Through therapy I learnt how to express myself assertively and respectfully, giving me the peace and relief I needed. In this chapter, I have merged 'Relationships Take Off' and 'Resource Maturity' to go through how these growth tools were helping me to put things into perspective and manage all forms of my relationships better.

Creating boundaries is a journey that I am still on. I am getting better at it each day and trying to stay consistent. There are times I fall off the wagon, but getting back up is what counts! Having boundaries has definitely created a healthier lifestyle for me. It means that I can focus on my needs first and then help others when I have the capacity to do so. The analogy of putting your oxygen mask on in an emergency before helping others speaks volumes. How can you truly help others when you are also struggling? There are times when things are pressing, but my therapist spoke to me about assessing how urgent a situation is with the other party to see whether my help is actually needed there and then. I am more at peace than I used to be, and I am more conscious of the relationships that are not serving me.

Closer to my 30th birthday it dawned on me that I still had not found that one person I wanted to spend the rest of my life with. I then started to reflect on the other things that I had achieved in my life and realised that despite not having that person, I was fulfilled. I turned 30 accepting that I was happy and enjoying my single season. Having a husband did not define my worth and I was whole on my own. Yes, it would be nice to find that person that adds (NOT brings) value to my life as long as it does not involve settling for anything less.

And so we take off using the tools we have learnt to create healthier relationships and better manage the relationships which are not serving us. With the use of these tools we should then ensure longevity by practising them and staying consistent with them – 'consistency' as you may have noticed, is a key word throughout this book. Having proper management of these tools is what I call 'Resource Maturity'.

In summary, I have learnt that not all relationships are meant to last forever and some relationships come for a season – to bring value to our lives for that season. I am therefore at peace with losing relationships that have run their course. I am learning how to better communicate with my family and friends – putting in boundaries where necessary. I have accepted that being single and happy is much better than being in an unfulfilling relationship and unhappy. In my single season, I have learnt to focus on the things that I have in my life that give me joy – so that when that special someone comes along, I can be in a better place to manage the relationship (none of us here are perfect – growing and learning to become better for ourselves and others is what counts). I am also implementing things that make me smile and living my life the best way I can. At the end of the day, prioritising my happiness is my number one goal and when I am happy, I know I can be the best version of myself to those in my life.

Thank you for taking your time to read through my relationships journey so far. It has been a journey and one that I am still on – as I mentioned, it is possible to fall off the wagon but always make sure you get back up again to keep that momentum going – trust me, it is so worth it! I wish you all the best in all forms of your relationships – may the ones that are working keep working, the ones that are going through the bumps get better, and the ones that you are looking to pursue blossom. Lastly, may you find healing for the relationships that have run their course.

Hebrews 10:24-25: 'And let us consider how we may spur one another on toward love and good deeds, not giving up meeting together, as some are in the habit of doing, but encouraging one another – and all the more as you see the day approaching'. Relationships are so important in this life. I am currently on a journey of building the best relationship that I can with God and through that journey, I am building healthier relationships with others. As mentioned, maintaining healthy relationships with others is about establishing boundaries and not just doing things because it will make someone else happy. Sometimes the things that make others happy are to our own detriment and may not always feel right in our spirit. Discernment has helped me in deciding whether something either feels right or wrong. For instance, when I feel that I am doing things for others out of obligation, as a result of pleasing people, I have noticed how various negative thoughts run through my mind. I believe that God does not want us to do things out of obligation for the sake of pleasing others when it feels wrong, but wants us to find joy in the things we do either for Him or others. I believe that taking care of our minds and souls is important in developing our relationships.

Relationships come in all forms, as mentioned at the start of this chapter. They allow us to share life with others, provide and receive support from others as well as build strong communities, so let us do whatever it takes to manage our relationships better!

CAREER – EXISTENCE

As mentioned in an earlier chapter, growing up, I was a people pleaser and part of this involved working hard at school to get good grades to please my parents. Much of this mentality also came from being brought up in a studious family. Both my parents are hard workers and high achievers. I watched my parents juggle as they raised us, my dad even managing to complete a PhD. Growing up, my parents rarely asked whether my homework had been done or whether I had done my revision for an exam – it was a given. Self-motivation and hard work were instilled in me from the age of eight. My family and I had left Malawi in 1996 to come to the UK, following my dad who was studying for his master's and then later on his PhD. Once he had completed his studies, we went back to Africa in the year 2000. We first went back to Malawi (where I was born) and then later travelled to Mozambique to live there. During our time in Mozambique, my sisters and I went to a boarding school in Swaziland whilst my younger brother continued school in Mozambique. It is at boarding school that I recall myself being motivated to do the best I could do in my school work without any parental supervision. The boarding school was extremely strict and it was the first time I witnessed children being beaten as punishment by teachers, even for the slightest mistakes. I remember being in class and getting 9/10 in a test and was extremely pleased with myself. I suddenly saw the teacher come towards me with a stick to strike me once on my hand for the one answer I got wrong. I was upset. As well as being brought up in a studious family, being at a strict boarding school also drove me to study hard so that I did not have to experience the pain of getting beaten for the slightest mistakes.

After several months at the boarding school, my parents decided to move the family to South Africa. There, my mum took on work as a teacher at the school my siblings and I were enrolled in. Although she was not my teacher, her being at the school put pressure on my siblings and I to do the best we could with our grades – not because my parents pressured us to, but because we did not want to let them down and cause any embarrassment. We aimed to be the highest achievers in our class and would compete with others in the aim of remaining position number one at the end of every school term. I remember studying extremely hard for all my exams just to be the best in the class, so much so that I made it to become a prefect.

In the year 2003, my parents made the decision for the family to move back to the UK. I was 11 years old at this time and really enjoyed reading which inspired me to want to become an author. I was so determined that I would write short stories and beg my family to read them. When I started secondary school, my favourite subject became maths, and I was good at it. Secondary school was the point in my life in which I really started to put a lot of thought into my future and, as mentioned in a previous chapter, had conversations with friends at the age of 15 that went like this:

'By the age of 25 I will be married, own a house, be in my dream career and be set for life.'

Again, I was planning things out so meticulously in my head, thinking that this was the standard route for a successful life. I remember being at school and making it my main focus to work hard and get the required grades that would get me to the next stage of my education and eventually my dream career. I was so set on becoming an economist from the age of 15 and was so sure that I would make this dream a reality.

During my A-levels I took subjects that would give me the best chance of eventually studying economics at university. I applied to the University of Southampton as my first choice. I received my A-level grades and my face dropped – I did not get the required grades to study economics at my preferred university. I felt as though my dreams had been crushed – just like that. I lost hope at that moment and told my family that I would take a gap year to decide what I want to do. At this point in my life, I did not have much confidence to explore other opportunities – I put so much focus and effort into my school work that I did not invest time looking into what else was out there. A gap year without a plan was therefore not the best option for me at this point in time. I spoke to my family about options and then decided to go through the clearing process. I thought about other courses that I wanted to study and accounting and finance came to mind – an accounting career became my new dream. I then started looking at universities that offered this course. I stumbled across Manchester Metropolitan University which offered the course and, luckily, I met the requirements. It meant that I would be a four-hour drive away from home but I was so excited for this new adventure and chapter of my life.

Manchester is a very exciting city with lots to do and explore. As a student there, I started settling in very quickly by making friends and getting to know the city. It was the first time that I felt true independence and I remember thinking, *I really needed this*. I got myself part-time agency work at the Manchester United stadium. Working was something that I always felt I needed to do as it gave me financial control which has always been important to me. Whilst working and enjoying university life with friends, I still had fire within me to work hard and achieve my goal of succeeding in an accounting career. A-levels had not gone the way I wanted them to so I was keen to now make this new 'dream' a reality.

I remember coming home after my final year at university waiting anxiously for my results. I had intense nightmares – the fear of a repeat of my A-level results made me incredibly tense. The letter finally came and I quickly opened it with shaky hands. The result was a first-class honours accounting and finance degree. I screamed and shouted with joy – I was so pleased that I erased all feelings of failure that came from receiving my A-level results in the past. My next step 'as it is written in the stars' was to get a job related to my degree.

After graduating, I moved back to my hometown of Reading and started confidently drawing up my CV. I smiled at my CV and applied to as many jobs as I could whilst also actively making appointments to see recruitment agents. In the meantime, I continued to work for a catering agency that I had worked for in Reading during the summer holidays whilst home from university. When I got a call to attend an interview for a tax assistant position at an accounting firm, I was very pleased. As soon as I received the news that I had passed the last stage of interviews for the position I was over the moon. My well-planned-out life was coming together, I thought to myself.

And this is how my career journey started. Was the 'dream' career really the dream though? In the next chapter, 'Career – Survival', I will take you through how I went into 'survival mode' whilst trying to convince myself that this was indeed the 'dream'.

Proverbs 16:9: 'The heart of man plans his way, but the Lord establishes his steps'. We can get so caught up in meticulously planning out our lives and this is exactly what I was doing as explained in this chapter. I was doing all the planning in my own strength and not seeking counsel or guidance. Instead of going by the motto 'God's got this', I was living by the motto of 'I've got this!'. At this point in time, I did not realise how exhausting it was thinking that I had to carry the load of my life plans, having only myself to rely on.

CAREER – SURVIVAL

In the last chapter, I wrote about how getting through the final stage of interviews for the tax assistant position gave me a feeling that 'my well-planned life was coming together'. However, after a year of working as a tax assistant and studying for my tax qualifications, I began to feel unhappy within my role. I thought to myself, *well, this can't be right*. I was on my way to my desired career journey so why was I so unhappy? As I continued working and studying, the feeling of unhappiness grew stronger and stronger. I then failed one of my tax exams with the option to retake it. The feeling that I had when I did not get my desired A-level grades started to creep in. I thought about how hard I had worked at university to become that high achiever again. I felt stuck knowing that I was unhappy at my job and failing the exam left me feeling even more discouraged. I didn't know what to do to shake this feeling. Did shaking this feeling mean leaving the job I so 'desired'? I thought long and hard and that is when things began to change... I gathered the courage and left my job with no back-up. I felt free but at the same time bogged down with worry. Luckily, I was still living with my parents but a voice in my head persisted: *you need to find a job quickly or else you will not succeed*. Adrenaline kicked in and I made it my full-time job to apply for jobs. It was very difficult as I did not know what my next steps would be, therefore

I applied for various finance/admin jobs. I was desperate to find a job but not to the point of accepting any job that came my way – the fear of being in the same unhappy position dawned on me.

I attended interviews and although I was called back for some of the roles I had interviewed for, they just did not feel right. I felt under pressure as I felt the need to find a job as quickly as possible but also had the fear of not wanting a repeat of the situation I had left. I had mixed emotions at this time. I then attended an interview at an accounting firm for a payroll administrator role. I got through both stages of the interview and accepted the offer after a month of being unemployed. I started the role not knowing exactly what to expect. I was 23 years old by this time and although I look back at how young I was, at that moment in time I felt like I needed to figure it all out there and then as time was ticking.

As I settled into my new situation, I found myself really enjoying the payroll administrator role. It was a global role which required liaising with various countries and coordinating payroll activities. The culture of the firm was great and embraced many things that I stood for. I started to learn a lot about myself whilst working in this role. I gave it my all and was truly appreciated by my colleagues for all my efforts. I received praise, but at this point in time I did not know how to respond to it or receive it as I felt that I was just doing what I was 'supposed' to do. Although I gave the job my all, deep down I knew I was going by the motto 'fake it till you make it'. 'Fake it till you make it' became the norm for me and is not something that I pondered on. I felt as though I constantly needed to prove myself.

As I continued with imposter syndrome – described as 'the persistent inability to believe that one's success is deserved or has been legitimately achieved as a result of one's own efforts or skills'[2] – I started to think about the direction I wanted to go in my career. As the department began to expand, more opportunities became available. I got involved in coordinating global payroll projects and training users on the systems – something I never would have seen myself doing. I was really enjoying the role and using my natural organisation and planning skills. Soon enough I became sure that I wanted to be a project manager but thought I did not have what it takes for such a role. I would regularly google the skills I needed for project management and although I had completed my PRINCE2 qualification, my lack of self-esteem was holding me back from stepping out. I then began to reflect on all the steps I had taken to get to the point I was at and the courage that it took. I knew there and then that I had to be bold and courageous and go for it if I really wanted it – and I did. I asked my manager if I could take up the opportunity of managing a project from beginning to end to see if this was truly what I wanted to do. It involved managing all stakeholders (internal and external), communicating project progress, ensuring timelines were met and numerous follow ups to ensure stakeholders were aware of critical timelines. My manager then assigned me my first project to run as a trial. I did not want to let her down and, most importantly, I really wanted this to work as I knew this was something I wanted to do and a career that I could really excel in due to the passion I had for it. Having imposter syndrome made me put in twice the work to make this a success. It worked and I ran the project successfully. My manager had confidence in me and allocated me more projects to manage.

As I ran the projects, I put many hours into my work to prove my worth. I would have so much on my to-do list but I kept on going and adding more onto the list. As mentioned in an earlier chapter, 'yes' was a word that came so naturally, meaning that I did not have any boundaries and this showed up in my work too. Although I had done enough to prove that I could do the job, I felt that I needed to continue to prove this by working over my contractual hours. Having no boundaries and imposter syndrome meant that I went into survival mode to keep things going which became exhausting. As mentioned in an earlier chapter, it is during lockdown that I sat still and could see the impact this was having on me mentally and physically. The pressure had become too much and I cracked. I could no longer contain the way I was feeling. Survival mode is a terrible feeling and, as mentioned, when we are not feeling the way we want to feel, we need to take the necessary steps that will help us get to where we want to be, which I call what? Yes, you got that right – 'SUCCESS'. I have learnt that having a successful life is not living and conforming to what society views as 'successful'. Success to me is living by what truly makes us happy by following our passions and allowing those passions to give us the best out of life. Once we find that passion, it is also ensuring that we manage that passion in the best way so that we benefit from it to live our best lives. I realised that an accounting/finance career was not for me and along the way I found something I was passionate about. I then needed to find a way of managing this passion better to live life the best way I could – imposter syndrome was definitely not the way to go. And this leads us into the next chapter, 'Career – Success'.

Proverbs 15:22: 'Without counsel, plans fail but with many advisers, they succeed'. Although I had found a career that I was passionate about, without guidance and advice, I struggled to manage it all, as shown in this chapter. Doing things in my own strength was not going the way I had planned – it was difficult and exhausting. At this point in time, I was so sure that I could figure it all out on my own. When I saw that things were not going the way I planned, I knew it was time to look for other solutions.

CAREER – SUCCESS

In the last chapter, I wrote about how I had found a career path that I was passionate about but then needed to find a way to manage it better. I put myself under a lot of pressure and I eventually cracked. After a couple of years of managing projects, I realised how the pressure was starting to affect me both mentally and physically. I started to break out in spots, I started having stomach pains and gut issues and was horrified when I realised that I was losing some hair! All this led to me feeling anxious and depressed.

As mentioned in an earlier chapter, I started therapy at the age of 29. During my therapy sessions, I spoke about how concerned I was with my working behaviours and the effect this was having on me mentally and physically. I felt as though I was 'a shell of myself' and those close to me could see this too. My therapist spoke to me about how I needed to prioritise my health and gave me ideas such as blocking time in my calendar to ensure that I prioritise my lunch breaks. This meant using my full contractual lunchtime to focus on out-of-work activities. It took me some time but I eventually started to take the time to really enjoy food away from my desk. I also took the time to enjoy my lunchtime outdoor walks, awakening all my senses to the views, the smells, and the sounds. It was truly refreshing. When I returned to my desk, I had more energy to continue on with my tasks and would log off at my contractual time. There were the odd days I would work a bit longer but I made it the norm to work what I was contracted to work. I also made it a priority to go to the GP for check-ups for the things I was concerned about.

With therapy, my self-esteem and sense of worth grew immensely. My therapist also asked me to reflect on the things I had achieved to date. As I began to reflect on all my successes I realised how deserving I was of opportunities and that I did not have to keep going above and beyond to prove my worth. This was a big step in my growth journey as someone who had always felt that I should be grateful for what I was given, no matter how little. Whilst gratitude is important, so is knowing your value. This started showing up in my work. I started to manage my workload better and declined requests that I could not manage. The fact that my co-workers respected this took me by surprise – setting these types of boundaries was so new to me. I started speaking up more and it felt more natural rather than the 'imposter syndrome' I had become so accustomed to. I surprised myself at how confidently I was respectfully challenging certain situations at work – I was truly empowered! It also made me realise that if I could not complete all tasks allocated to me in that given time, therefore affecting me mentally and physically, then something had to change. When I first started managing projects, working extra hours to prove myself was the norm. I realised that I had done enough to show my worth and began to prioritise looking after myself.

As my confidence grew, I started to demand more at work, backed up by the research I did to prove my worth. From the research, I found that I deserved more from my role than I could have previously imagined. When the company could not meet requests I considered to be fair, my self-worth made me realise that it was time to move on. At this point, I had been at the firm for almost seven years and had just turned 30. I was grateful for the growth this role had given me both personally and professionally but also felt that I was ready for the next challenge in my career. I then started looking into other roles still on the mindset of progressing my project management career. I applied and interviewed for a project manager role at a software company and accepted the offer.

The job offer came through three days after my 30th birthday – to me this was a big sign for a new and exciting chapter of my life. I had learnt so much about myself and it was the first time that I genuinely felt that this was what I wanted for my career. I felt 'successful' and not because I was following society's idea of success but because I felt happy within myself. I had taken the steps to gain confidence in my abilities and worth without feeling the need to prove myself by going above and beyond.

As mentioned in an earlier chapter, when we continue to use the tools we have gained to become better versions of ourselves, we then have to learn to become consistent so that it becomes a lifestyle. Therapy had given me the tools I needed to reach a stage in which I felt empowered and it was my job to continue using these tools with consistency. This leads us into the next chapter, 'Career – Take Off and Resource Maturity'.

Proverbs 19:21: 'Many are the plans in the mind of a man, but it is the purpose of the Lord that will stand'. Therapy has definitely helped me in managing myself better and so does leaning on God. Leaning on God gives me permission to do what I can and leave the rest to Him by surrendering. This is what God wants us to do and if God does not want us to worry or fear because He's got this, then who am I to continue bringing fear and worry upon myself? I believe that He is working things out for my good and through spending time with him, I see things a lot more clearly. I listen when something doesn't feel right and know that it is a sign. I strongly believe that God has a purpose for my life and through spending time with Him, I feel like I am getting closer to it each day. I am no longer going by the motto 'I've got this' but instead 'God's got this'. This brings me so much peace knowing that I do not have to carry the heavy load alone.

CAREER – TAKE OFF AND RESOURCE MATURITY

In the last chapter, I wrote about how I started therapy and how this helped me manage my career and make decisions that were better for me mentally and physically.

I started working at the software company as a project manager in February 2022 which is where my career in project management really took off. I was then promoted to senior project manager in September 2023, exploring ways to further enhance my leadership skills. I was also trusted by my manager to lead on more complex projects and have been given the opportunity to showcase my skill through various opportunities. Through this journey, I learnt to trust myself and to always remember how valuable I am – that is MY responsibility. I grew as a person and my roles have pushed me out of my comfort zone which is where I have seen the most growth within myself. Therapy has definitely been a big part in this transformation allowing me to 'take off' using the tools I have learnt and ensuring longevity by staying consistent. Having proper management of these tools is what I call 'Resource Maturity'. I have learnt that no matter how much we try to 'fake it till we make it', it will eventually catch up with us if this is our sole method, therefore it is best to really work through any insecurities to truly succeed. Working through the insecurities allows us to show up as our true authentic selves, which feels so much easier and natural.

I have also learnt that life is not rigid and no matter how much we plan it, it does not always go our way. I have learnt to be resilient, accept challenges and move my plans around, therefore if plan 'A' fails – that does not make me a failure. Sometimes in life, plan 'A' was not meant to be, but plans 'B – Z' have so much more to offer.

I am still on my career journey discovering new things each day, making plans but knowing that it is okay if plans change. My outlook on life and my career has definitely grown and matured. There is no 'standard' way to do it and looking back on my path and hearing the experiences of others, I see that there are countless ways to succeed in life and success can look different to various people. In terms of career, I now realise that success for me is not just about doing a job I felt I was 'supposed' to do per my plan, but doing a job that I am passionate about and a job that fulfils me, gives me purpose and makes me happy – there may be unfulfilling days but most days should bring joy.

Throughout my career journey, I realised that I was doing everything through my own strength and making plans without guidance and counsel. I will discuss this more in my spirituality chapters, as mentioned in the introduction. I have now come to the conclusion that my eternal confidence lies in God. 2 Timothy 1:7 reads 'For the spirit God gave us does not make us timid, but gives us power, love and self-discipline'. Without this eternal confidence from God, I cannot sustain everything in my own strength as it eventually runs out. I have experienced that picking myself back up from life's challenges without help from God is the most difficult thing.

Thank you for taking your time to go through my career journey with me. I wish you all the best in your career journey and the steps you are taking to get to wherever you want to be. If it genuinely makes you happy then take the chance! It will be worth it!

Proverbs 16:3 reads 'Commit to the Lord whatever you do and he will establish your plans'. As mentioned, I have noticed that involving God in the plans I make provides me with the comfort and reassurance that I do not have to figure it out on my own. As well as seeking guidance from the people I trust, I have realised that having God as my first point of call is the most peaceful feeling. The journey to faith and believing that God can carry the load if I let Him is one that I certainly struggled with. In the next chapter, I will take you through my spiritual journey so, as you may have guessed, the next chapter will be 'Spirituality – Existence'.

SPIRITUALITY – EXISTENCE

My parents raised my siblings and I in the Christian faith. My first memory of going to church was when I was four years old and we had just arrived in the UK (the family went to church in Malawi before this, but I have no recollection). With Malawi being a former British colony, my parents adopted the Anglican tradition and we attended a local Anglican church in the UK. When I returned to Africa and lived in various countries, we continued to attend Anglican churches there.

When I was a child, I enjoyed Sunday school and receiving treats after the church service. I enjoyed listening to the biblical stories as well as the arts and crafts during the Sunday school sessions. When I came back to the UK at the age of 11, my family and I went back to attending our local Anglican church. I enjoyed the music and singing hymns in a high-pitched voice. However, I eventually felt that I was not getting much from the preaching and felt it did not relate to my circumstances. At the age of 16, my interest in going to our local Anglican church gradually shifted. I always cherished my faith for giving me hope and belief in something higher. That's why, when I received invitations to attend various types of churches, I accepted the offers. I particularly enjoyed attending Pentecostal churches which I found very lively and a nice change.

When I went to university, I took it upon myself to find a church. Although I did not attend regularly, it was a nice feeling when I did as I still felt connected to my faith. However, there were many moments I felt disconnected – I did not pray or read the Bible regularly which meant there were high and low moments in my spiritual journey. When I finished university, I went back to my hometown (Reading) and attended some services at the local Anglican church. As life started 'lifing' and adulting became real, I realised again that I had no connection with the preaching and felt that I needed something more relatable to the situations I was going through at that point in my life. I stopped going to church altogether. By this time my sister was living in Oxford and when I would travel from Reading at the weekend to see her, I started to attend the Pentecostal church that she attended. I really started to enjoy the church as most of the preaching was relevant to the situations I was facing in my life. I found it refreshing that I would try on most Sundays to attend the church. From there, I started to feel more spiritually connected to my faith. Before, I would occasionally go to church, occasionally pray and occasionally read the Bible, but I was now becoming more intentional about my faith.

However, after some time of attending the church in Oxford and after facing some challenges in life, I began to question my faith. At this point in time I was 23 years old. I felt as though life was not going the way I wanted and I questioned that. I then decided to stop going to church altogether again. I slowly drifted from all the connections that I had to my faith and after some time I started to feel lost. I was down and lacked the comfort of having hope and belief in something higher than myself. My faith had been the thing I would turn to when I felt internally alone and drifting away from it brought a feeling of loneliness. I felt conflicted as I was eager to get answers to the questions I had but, at the same time, I was scared of pulling away from my faith completely.

The questions I had came from listening to various people's interpretations of the Bible. I was also facing life challenges that had me wondering whether God had forgotten about me. I also had some friends who were non-believers and would ask me questions that I could not give answers to, bringing about more questions. As this continued, the conflict within me grew. I hated having this feeling of needing answers, being questioned and not knowing what to believe anymore yet at the same time feeling lost without my faith.

Deuteronomy 31:6 reads 'Be strong and courageous. Do not fear or be in dread of them, for it is the Lord your God who goes with you. He will not leave you or forsake you'. At this point in my life, I could feel myself drifting further away from my faith and God. This verse is a reminder that even during those moments in which we drift away from God, He is always there waiting for us to come back to Him. The next chapter is 'Spirituality – Survival' in which I will go deeper into the feeling of being lost in my faith and losing hope in certain areas of my life.

SPIRITUALITY – SURVIVAL AND SUCCESS

In the last chapter I wrote about feeling conflicted about needing answers to questions I had about my faith but also the fear of losing my faith and feeling lost without it. At this point in my life, I felt that things were not going to plan and, as mentioned, I felt as though God had forgotten about me. The career path I had dreamed of was not working out, my dreams of having a husband and starting a family were not coming to fruition. I had a lot of questions that I felt I needed answers to. In this chapter, I have combined Spirituality Survival and Spirituality Success.

After some time of drifting away from church, reading the Bible, praying and overall intentional faith, I started to feel alone. Although surrounded by people, there were certain things that I did not feel comfortable sharing and thought that people would not understand. I felt empty and lost. As mentioned in earlier chapters, survival mode in my relationships meant I had no boundaries, with 'yes' being my default answer. This was the same situation in my career life in which I was struggling with imposter syndrome and felt as though I needed to be that same 'yes' person to prove my worth. All of this, without hope and faith, was a struggle. I felt stuck.

I hated feeling this way and knew I needed something to lift my spirits. I then decided to go back to church. Not because I had all my questions answered but because I missed having hope and faith. I then started to attend various churches, Sunday after Sunday, seeking connection. I went back to the church in Oxford but the distance made it difficult to attend every Sunday. I eventually stopped and continued to scout churches in Reading. Whilst in Oxford, I had also attended Hillsong church which is a charismatic Christian non-denominational megachurch – I enjoyed the service. I heard that there was also a Hillsong Guildford church, so I started to attend as it was easier to get to from Reading. The first service I attended there was beyond amazing. The message, as well as the worship, gave me goosebumps. It was very relatable and I felt at peace being there. The people I met there were also very friendly and welcoming. I walked out of the service feeling as though a weight had been lifted off of my shoulders. I felt as though I had experienced a spiritual awakening.

There were eventually plans to open a Hillsong Reading church and a friend of mine also started a Hillsong Reading connect group. This was a space for people of a similar age group to get together, hang out, talk about faith and any relatable challenges. I found this refreshing. Before the Covid-19 pandemic, the Reading church opened up. I attended regularly and volunteered to be part of the welcome team which I really enjoyed. When the pandemic hit and the country went into lockdown, all of this stopped and everything went online. During this time, I did not attend the online services much, however I would listen to other sermons, which is when my love for the preaching of Pastor Sarah Jakes Roberts started. I found it so relatable that I would feel goosebumps anytime I tuned in.

As mentioned in previous chapters, lockdown and the pandemic is the time I started to realise how various aspects of life had been affecting me mentally and physically which led me into seeking therapy. Although I was being more intentional about my faith and felt more connected, I also felt I needed an integration of therapy and spirituality to help me process the situations I was going through. Spirituality was giving me hope and belief that there are seasons for everything in life. It was also giving me faith that there is a higher power I can call upon to get me through any situation. Therapy was giving me the tools to navigate each season. I also loved how Sarah Jakes Roberts would speak openly about therapy, something that, from my experience, had been frowned upon within the faith community. The way I see it now is that in the same way a believer goes to the hospital when they are physically ill, they should by all means seek therapy for mental and emotional healing.

I can testify that both therapy and faith have helped me get through the day-to-day challenges of life. In October 2021, when my best friend sadly passed away at the age of 29, it was a combination of my faith and the tools I was learning in therapy that got me through. It was extremely tough and ultimately, I can only thank God for helping me process it up until this day. And so, with that said, I want to dedicate this chapter to my best friend Halima:

> 'Thank you for being the best sister friend a person could ever wish for. I thank God for bringing you into my life and allowing me to share so many wonderful moments with you. Thank you for understanding me and bringing so much joy into my life. Thank you for the many moments of uncontrollable laughter in which our stomachs would hurt – even in public where people would stare. Thank you for the moments of comfortable silence and for the moments we allowed ourselves to be vulnerable. Thank you for always calling me to check up on me and to hear the mundane details of my day – no matter how boring you would always listen. Thank you for the many hours we would spend talking about so many things – the good, the bad, the ugly, the random. I always laugh at the similarities we shared – 100% my personal person. Thank you for being weird with me. Thank you for the inside jokes we built up over the years. Thank you for being there. I can only hope and pray that you felt the same efforts and friendship from me as I did from you. A young, gorgeous and beautiful soul (inside and out) with so much love to give – may you keep shining, my angel. I miss you each and every day. I will continue to cherish and hold onto the awesome memories until we meet again… love you forever and always xxx'

Romans 15:13 reads 'May the God of hope fill you with joy and peace as you trust in him so that you may overflow with hope by the power of the holy spirit'. With hope and faith, I know that this is not the end. Trusting in God has definitely given me peace in challenging situations and I am grateful that by this point in time I was at a place in which I wanted to draw closer to God again. As mentioned in the previous chapter, God never leaves us or forsakes us and when we are ready, He is waiting for us to come back and continue building a relationship with Him. Going through traumatic experiences is part of human nature. We often ask ourselves that, if there is a God, why would he allow these traumatic experiences to occur. Through reading the Bible I have gained an understanding that traumatic experiences were not part of God's initial plan.

I understand that God's love runs deep, and through my challenging experiences I have experienced joy and peace by connecting and spending time with Him.

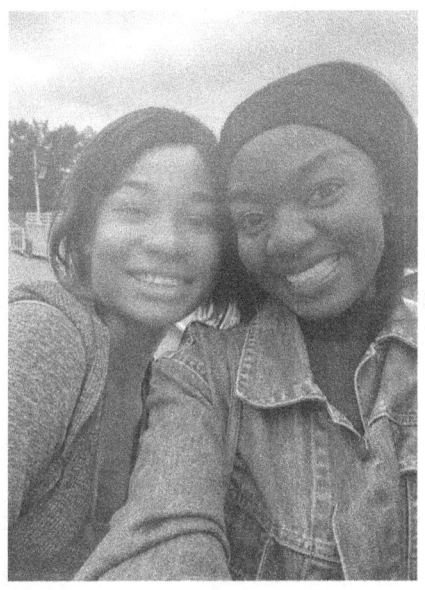

Love you forever and always.

In the next chapter 'Spirituality – Take Off and Resource Maturity' I will take you through how I am constantly learning through faith and the tools I have gained in therapy to become a better version of myself. As said before, consistency is key and when we fall, we can always get back up again – no one is perfect!

SPIRITUALITY – TAKE OFF AND RESOURCE MATURITY

In the last chapter, I wrote about how both spirituality and therapy were helping me navigate the day-to-day challenges of life. I mentioned that although not all my questions regarding my faith had been answered, I persisted with going back to church and finding a church that best met my needs – I continued attending Hillsong Reading church and just love how it fulfils me spiritually to this day. I am also persisting with being more intentional about my faith.

As for my questions, I began to read the Bible, seek interpretation (as well as ask those who had studied it) and pray on it rather than pay too much attention to the many views I'd hear. There are so many views in this world that can sway us in various directions. Ultimately, I believe that Christianity is based on each individual's relationship with God, which may look different from person to person. That is the reason I find it difficult to see when people place judgement on others for not living to their standard of the 'Christian way'. Who are we to judge at the end of the day?

My spiritual journey has been one with ups and downs, but I arrived at a place where I feel at peace with it. There are steps that I am taking and would like to take to strengthen my relationship with God and I am constantly learning each day. As mentioned in earlier chapters, none of us are perfect but doing the work to become better versions of ourselves is what counts.

I have witnessed many miraculous moments in my life that I know did not happen by chance. There are moments in which I prayed for something and saw it come to fruition and there are moments the things I prayed for did not come to pass. One thing I do believe is that for some of those things that did not come to pass – God had/has something better in mind. I am a strong believer that if you work hard at something and pray to God for guidance, trusting Him, it will come your way (maybe not always in the way you planned it, but in a better version). I also believe that things happen for a reason. Although things did not work out the way I had planned, I believe God was/is preparing better – my job is to remain patient and listen to signs from God by spending time with Him through worship, prayer and reading the Bible. When things did not work out the way I planned, I felt as though God had forgotten about me (I still have those moments from time to time), however, I am generally at peace with where I am in life. God is revealing my purpose to me each day and I have seen miraculous events happen right before my eyes. He is merging various aspects of my life and removing any distractions to ensure I can fully walk with Him to where He is leading me. I am gladly and faithfully following. It has been scary on occasions and sometimes lonely, but I am truly at a place where I believe that doing life with God is the best decision I have ever made!

I am grateful for all the things God has brought into my life to this day as mentioned in earlier chapters – things that bring me joy. I am also happy to have my faith to turn to through the ups and downs of life. When I have those moments in which I feel God has forgotten about me, I stay reminded that I am seeking and waiting on God for the big plans He has for me – being conscious that I also have to do the work and watch out for the signs by leaning in and listening to what God is telling me. This verse gives me joy: '"For I know the plans I have for you," declares the Lord, "plans to prosper you and not to harm you, plans to give you a hope and a future."' — Jeremiah 29:11.

As I look ahead and into the future, I pray it is one full of joy and so many blessings. I pray for growth in various areas of life as well as patience and wisdom. I pray that we stay reminded to show kindness and grace to one another. This world is a world full of surprises, and kindness is so simple!

1 Peter 5:7 reads 'Cast all your anxiety on him because he cares for you'. It gives me great joy that God does not want us to live a life of anxiety or fear. God wants us to be confident in Him and to know that through Him all things are possible. I have realised that having fear and anxiety means doubting God and what He can do in your life. There is such a peaceful and calm feeling I receive from this knowing that I don't have to carry the weight of fear and anxiety on my shoulders, and I can choose to live a life free from it by believing and trusting

in God. As a person who easily gets anxious and worries, this has helped me in so many situations.

Thank you for going through my spirituality journey with me. In the next chapter, I will be moving onto the next topic – Health (Mental and Physical). The next chapter will be 'Health – Existence'.

HEALTH – EXISTENCE

Taking care of our bodies and mind should be our number one priority because it is our bodies and minds that help us to function in our day-to-day. However, sometimes the things that are 'bad' for us can often seem so good in the moment. From what I have experienced, that eventually wears off. This topic of my life journey in the form of a business lifecycle is Health. My health (both mental and physical) were touched upon in previous chapters (Relationships – Survival and Career – Success) therefore this will serve as a summary with a specific focus on health.

During my youth, health and self-care were not a priority to me. With regards to physical health, the only exercise I would do was during PE classes and when playing games with friends on the playground. Having a sweet tooth meant I would consume so much junk food without thinking about the long-term effects it could have on my health. During secondary school, I remember walking to and from school and would stop at the corner shop to buy junk food for the journey – Haribo sweets being my choice for breakfast. I was not very keen on extra-curricular activities and so didn't take part in any sports.

As for my mental health, this was something that was not talked about at this point in my life. It is not something that occurred to me and is not something that I thought about. I would carry on with my day-to-day activities without thinking about how certain situations within my family, friendships and various other relationships affected me.

Looking back at my childhood, I recognise the negative effects of failing to prioritise my mental and physical health. I can remember feeling this way from the age of 11. My family and I had just moved back to the UK from South Africa after having been in Africa for three years. At this point in time, I was very much in my own shell. I did not express myself and kept all my feelings to myself. I became withdrawn and often felt isolated from others around me which made it difficult to engage and make friends. Although I did make friends I never spoke about the things that bothered me.

As I grew older, I continued on with eating habits that I deem as bad when I look back. I also continued getting on with life and not really considering how situations in life were affecting me mentally as mental health was not really a 'thing' in my community. As mentioned in earlier chapters, there are various aspects of life that can affect us mentally and oftentimes it can be a ripple effect. For example, not managing relationships in the best way possible can have an effect on your career, spiritual wellness or health.

When I finished university and went back to my hometown in the hopes of starting my 'dream' life, I was crushed when certain things were not going the way I planned as you would have read in previous chapters (Relationships – Survival, Career – Survival and Spirituality – Survival and Success). Although I did not realise it initially, this affected me mentally and physically. Physically, because of the stress I put myself under trying to manage life, which had a negative impact on my body. I was also mentally affected by the stress and did not have the tools to help me manage my emotions. Without these tools, I went into survival mode doing whatever I could to keep my life moving. Survival mode is definitely not a good feeling.

Winter is normally a time my mental and physical health suffer most. During this season, I ensure that I stay prepared by focusing and staying consistent with the following:

1. Being consistent with running at least three times a week mixing this with any other form of exercise two times a week.
2. Daily ten-minute walks (ideally in the morning).
3. Being intentional with gratitude and deep breathing.
4. Being consistent with my morning Bible devotions using the 'YouVersion' bible app.[11]
5. Drinking more water (I find it hard to drink cold water in the winter so warm water is my go-to).

Corinthians 3:16 reads 'Do you not know that you are God's temple and that God's spirit dwells in you?'. This verse provides me with comfort and is a reminder of how important it is for me to look after myself, mentally, physically and spiritually. As mentioned previously, God's intention is for us to live a life free from anxiety and fear and letting these feelings manifest has a huge impact on our mental health. To me, this verse also means that as well as looking after our minds, God also wants us to look after our bodies and souls. I don't know about you but when all these three elements are healthy, I definitely feel great within myself. Maintaining all three takes intention.

In the next chapter, 'Health – Survival and Success', I will take you through how I went into survival mode and the impact this had on my health. I will also take you through how I overcame being in the state of survival mode and the tools I used to get me there – success.

HEALTH – SURVIVAL AND SUCCESS

In the last chapter, I wrote about how my approach to health started on a 'not so good note' – both mentally and physically. I also referenced earlier chapters, in which I wrote about how various areas of my life were having an impact on my health. Without having the tools to manage my mental health, I went into survival mode to keep things moving which had an effect on my physical health. This is because I would often use junk food to cover up negative feelings of having a bad day – it became so comforting. There were also times that I would get stomach cramps from a continual amount of anxiety and stress which led to me breaking out in spots, therefore again impacting my mental health.

It was a cycle that I wanted to break free from. This is when I began to seek therapy as mentioned in earlier chapters. Therapy helped me work on my relationships and career, giving me the tools to best manage these areas. This started to ease the stress and anxiety I was experiencing in the day-to-day of trying to manage these areas under survival mode. Spiritual healing also played a big part in this. As I have mentioned before, working through all these areas of my life is still a work in progress, but being aware and conscious of when I am falling off and in need of a refill is great progress to me!

I paused therapy in June 2023 after having started in March 2021. I decided to stop because I could see progress within myself, and others could too – it was a great feeling receiving compliments of the positive change people could see in me. When I am in need of a re-fill, I go back to having my therapy sessions and find a therapist that best meets my needs. As well as therapy, other tools that keep me reminded of the journey I am on are:

- Continuing with attending church – enjoying the community and being more intentional with my faith.
- Following YouTubers who are on a similar journey to me and who speak about things that inspire me to do better.
- Joining a community of people who are health-conscious (and like to make it fun at the same time).
- Listening to podcasts that inspire me.

With all of the above, I am continuing to see an improvement within myself and I know I have to stay consistent and disciplined with this lifestyle to prevent myself from falling back into my old ways. This progress is what I call 'success' – becoming self-aware and choosing the 'better' ways to manage any setbacks. I definitely have my 'bad' days in which I feel anxious, stressed and depressed but having a self-care toolkit that works for me is definitely handy on such days – my personal self-care toolkit can be found at the end of this book. Sometimes it takes giving yourself permission to feel the way you do when you have those 'bad days' but knowing that you cannot prolong that feeling and you eventually need to snap out of it. Once you snap out of it you can then get back on track to that 'feel-good' feeling by choosing the things that are good for you mentally and physically. I am also grateful to have therapy as a tool to use when I feel I am in need of it.

Psalms 46:5 reads 'God is within her, she will not fall; God will help her at break of day'. This verse is comforting and as mentioned many times before, leaning on God's strength encourages me to never give up and keep going. It encourages me to continue looking after my body, mind and soul knowing that I can always rely on God as my strength and helper. Leaning into God's word and inviting Him into my daily life is something that I need to do to ensure that I am doing okay mentally, physically and spiritually so that when it all becomes too much, I can surrender it all to God and take the break that I need to.

I hope that you are taking all the necessary steps to prioritise your health and are doing the things that are good for you both mentally and physically. Remember 'health is wealth' and giving your mind, soul and body the best fighting chance is the best gift you can give to yourself! The next chapter of this book is 'Health – Take Off and Resource Maturity'.

HEALTH – TAKE OFF AND RESOURCE MATURITY

In the previous chapter, I wrote about ways in which I started to prioritise my health mentally, physically and spiritually. I also mentioned the tools I used to assist me with this. I am still on this journey but what I do know so far is that I want to carry on with the habits I have started and continue being consistent and disciplined with them. These can be found in the 'Self-Care Toolkit' section of this book which you will find at the end of the book. There are times I am hard on myself for not reaching the targets I set, so this is something I want to stop doing. I want to give myself more grace – work hard to achieve my goals but also schedule time to rest and reset. Resetting will allow me to reflect on the areas in which I need a refill and work out the tools I need for that – as they say, 'you cannot pour from an empty cup!'. There are seasons in which I start to feel overwhelmed. At the start of each year, I usually start by setting myself goals and pushing myself to keep up with all of them, beating myself up on the days and times I do not meet my targets. This is a sign to me that I need a reset and reflect on the goals I had set myself and break them down into achievable tasks. This is where my 12-week year planning comes into place. I tend to start using the 12-week year to plan my goals so that I feel less overwhelmed. More information about the 12-week year can be found in the 'A Hack to Managing the To-do Lists of Life' section at the end of the book.[3]

I am definitely keen to keep up with a healthier diet whilst making room for treats here and there. As mentioned in my earlier chapters, I have a sweet tooth and crave all things sweet. Although I have started replacing the bad sugars with healthier options, I am continuously working on becoming more consistent and disciplined.

As well as my physical and mental health, I am also becoming more intentional about my faith to improve my overall spiritual wellness. This includes taking time to really understand where I am spiritually by spending more time with God. This includes prioritising time in my day to connect with God by reading my Bible, praying and worshiping Him. From the past, I have seen that when I am in a good place spiritually, I get that 'feel-good' feeling.

I would like to continue working on ways to become a better version of myself where I am competing with nobody else but me!

Philippians 4:6-8 reads 'Do not be anxious about anything, but in everything by prayer supplication with thanksgiving let your requests be made known to God. And the peace of God which surpasses all understanding, will guard your hearts and your minds in Christ Jesus. Finally, brothers, whatever is true, whatever is honourable, whatever is just, whatever is pure, whatever is lovely, whatever is commendable, if there is any excellence, if there is anything worthy of praise, think about these things'. This verse sums up where I am at with my life. As an over-thinker and as someone who easily gets anxious, this verse is a true life-saver. Hearing that I do not have to let anxiety rule my life and that I can give it all to God in prayer is the best thing ever. This is the comfort that prayer to God has offered me through the ups and downs of life. It gives me so much peace.

FINANCES – EXISTENCE AND SURVIVAL

Growing up, finances did not mean a thing to me. I would ask for things from my parents without having any concept of the price. I did not understand it when my mum would walk into a shop keen to compare the price of an item from one store to the next to make sure she was getting the best bargain. I did not understand being told, 'No, there is food at home,' when all I longed for was a scrumptious McDonald's burger.

I got my first job at the age of 16. I was over the moon when I received the job offer just a few hours after being interviewed for the position. My first job was at a Clarks baggage store which sold handbags and luggage. Receiving my first pay check felt great! I had no responsibilities therefore could spend the money on anything I wanted. I had no concept of savings. Even though I had witnessed the idea of bargaining for the best deals, this did not stick with me. I would head into town with money in my bank account, and without a plan would go into shops buying anything I could get my hands on. At this point in time, I was not a savvy buyer. I would buy items of low quality and hoard them. One thing that I do commend myself for was using some of my money to go towards my driving lessons. Other than that, my money management skills were extremely poor.

At the age of 18, I went to university. As mentioned in the 'Career' chapter of this book, I had a part-time agency job at the Manchester United stadium. I also mentioned that having a job and earning was something I felt I needed to do as it gave me financial control. During my holidays from university, I also signed up with a catering agency in my hometown Reading which allowed me to earn extra money. Although I had some money coming in on top of my student loan, my money management skills had not changed. As soon as I received an income, I would spend my money on either clothes or food. As mentioned, the clothes I bought were of a very poor quality and therefore did not last long – I was very much into fast fashion at this point.

After I graduated from university and started working full time, I was still living at home with my parents. At this point in time, I was in my early 20s. Since I was working full time, I contributed towards the household bills, however, the rest of the money I received was still being managed poorly and I had no concept of investing money for the future. As I started to aspire for the things that I wanted in life such as buying a house and being financially stable, I knew that this mentality had to change, and I had to become more intentional about managing my money better. Talking about money made me feel uncomfortable which is another mentality I knew I had to change.

The two main concepts I had about money were to spend it on low quality items and give it out to whoever asked me for it (refer to my people pleasing ways in previous chapters). These two concepts started to become dangerous territory. Spending my money on low quality items rather than high quality items made me feel as though I was using my money better – definitely not in the long-term! I looked at the price of high-quality items and would turn my head away. I also denied myself of self-care experiences such as holidays, spa trips – my thought at the time was that they were too expensive and unnecessary. Some would say that I was being 'stingy' with my money even though I was not managing it well either. The other concept, which was dangerous territory, was giving my money out to whoever asked me for it. As mentioned, I did not like to talk about money, therefore if I lent someone money and did not receive it back, I would write off the money and continue lending it to them whilst writing it off each time.

The feeling of being uncomfortable talking about money followed me into my work life. I found it difficult to negotiate salaries during job interviews and at pay reviews. I would simply take what was on offer and was just grateful to have a job. I also took this same mentality into relationships. Whether it be a platonic relationship or a romantic relationship, I had no issue spending money on others but would shy away from others spending money on me. It somehow made me feel guilty. I grew up listening to people misquote the Bible by saying 'money is the root of all evil'. Being a people pleaser, as well as taking this misquote to heart, made me feel the need to give out money whenever someone asked me for it – regardless of how much money I had for myself. Once I started studying the Bible for myself I came across 1 Timothy 6:10 which actually reads 'For the love of money is a root of all kinds of evil'. I then understood that it is that 'love' of money that can lead to evil. Having money, managing it well and talking about money is not evil.

In my mid-20s, I could see that a combination of these things were setting me back in my finances. I wanted more in terms of my finances, but I was not taking the necessary actions to help my finances grow. I felt stuck in the sense that I wanted more for my life but felt unsure of where to start. I was in survival mode, continuing to mismanage my finances whilst still wanting so much more for my life.

In the next chapter 'Finances – Success', I will take you through the steps I took to help me better manage my finances to achieve my goals and how I achieved success.

FINANCES – SUCCESS

In the previous chapter, I wrote about how mismanaging my finances was preventing me from financial breakthrough. I also talked about how approaching my finances in this way made me feel stuck as I wanted more for my life. In my mid-20s I became serious about getting onto the property ladder and owning a house. As mentioned in previous chapters, I was disappointed when a husband had not come along in the hopes and dreams that we would come together and purchase a home. I then started looking into options. During this time, I had moved out of my parents' house and was renting. I would look at house prices and compare this to the money I had saved up over the years – my poor money management meant I had very little and I was nowhere close to getting a deposit for a house. My sister was living in Oxford at this point, and was renting a place there. We started having conversations about house ownership as we were both at a stage in our lives where we wanted a place of our own. We discussed our options and decided we would put our finances together and buy a house together.

We also discussed the sacrifices we would need to make if we really wanted this. The first step was to move back in with our parents, therefore giving up the places we were renting, which worked really well. We moved back into our parents' house, as mentioned in the introduction of this book. We contributed to household bills and at the same time we managed to save up tirelessly with the goal of buying our first home. Although my money management skills were still not great, there were some sacrifices I made to ensure that my sister and I hit our saving goals to buy a house. As a people pleaser, I was still in the habit of lending money to anyone who asked for it and I had very poor budgeting skills. Being generous with money is definitely a great thing, however, being responsible with money is equally as important. 2 Corinthians 9:6 reads 'Remember this: Whoever sows sparingly will also reap sparingly' and whoever sows generously will also reap generously'. This verse to me means that there needs to be a balance. It is a good thing to be helpful and to give generously when you have the money, however if you give and spend money irresponsibly you will reap sparingly.

I also continued to spend my money on eating out and invaluable items. My sister is really good at managing her money so we spoke about tips for better money management. She had a system for budgeting for the month to ensure she was not overspending in certain areas. She also made and carried lunch to work, which helped elevate her savings. I decided to put the same habits into place – they were hard at first but I began to adopt them. Sacrifices have to be made when we are serious about reaching our goals! I continued with these sacrifices which eventually led to me becoming a homeowner at the age of 27. My sister and I were so thrilled. Although my faith was at a rocky place at this point in time, God definitely played a huge role. I say this because I still had some difficulties in money management which I knew I needed to continue to work on. Despite this, we managed to get the house we wanted and the process was extremely smooth for us. During the process, my sister and I heard about the many horror stories that people had experienced, some involving the house falling through. I am so grateful to God for guiding my sister and I through the process.

As mentioned in the introduction, my sister and I moved into the house just before the Covid pandemic and lockdown. In various chapters of this book, I have mentioned how lockdown is a time that made me reflect on my mental health and people pleasing ways. People pleasing was a factor that was setting me back in wisely managing my finances as I felt the need to give and lend money even when I did not have it to give. Going to therapy helped me to work through these feelings. Therapy also gave me the confidence I needed to ask for what I deserved at my workplace. I knew that I also had to become comfortable with talking about money to achieve this. As mentioned in my career chapter, I started to ask for what I deserved, which included my salary. This definitely helped me to level up my finances. Through these methods I felt 'successful'. Not just because of the money increase, which was definitely a blessing, but because I was developing the tools I needed to help me manage my finances better. As mentioned throughout this book, taking the necessary steps that will help us get to where we want to be is what I call

'SUCCESS', therefore living in a way where fear, doubt, worry and lack of confidence are not holding us back from where we want to be. As I have mentioned, God's intention is for us to live a life free from these things so why carry the load? No one said it will be easy, but it is definitely worth it!

Deuteronomy 8:18 NIV reads 'But remember the Lord your God, for it is he who gives you the ability to produce wealth, and so confirms his covenant, which he swore to your ancestors, as it is today'. This verse to me means that God is the source of my finances. Through my relationship with Him and through trusting Him, I have definitely seen breakthroughs in my finances. Trusting also means giving to others when I am able to, allowing God to continue to be a blessing in my life as well as a blessing to others.

FINANCES – TAKE OFF AND RESOURCE MATURITY

In the previous chapter, I wrote about the methods that I started using to help me manage my finances better. I now had to focus on making these methods a lifestyle to ensure that I continued on my journey of financial growth. As mentioned in the chapters of this book, this is what I call 'Take Off and Resource Maturity'.

Reaching the age of 30, my finances were in a much better place. Therapy and growing my relationship with God were two key methods that had helped me. I am still on this journey and still have hiccups along the way, but I have found that having discipline in this area has helped me continue to manage my finances in a healthy way. I am discovering and learning new ways to grow my finances each day. There are so many ideas in this world that are presented to us as an encouragement to grow our finances, also known as 'side hustles' that can grow into businesses. Having so many ideas can often feel overwhelming. I have now reached the stage in my spiritual journey where I pray about the ideas that are presented to me and through prayer, I am guided through the best direction to take, which is felt by the peace I receive. Growing our finances also comes with putting in the work which is very vital.

As mentioned in previous chapters, doing things in my own strength was a struggle and very challenging. Trusting God and surrendering to Him when my strength runs out is the biggest relief. Trusting in God requires me to have the understanding that God's plans are bigger than the plans I have for myself. This can sometimes lead to disappointment, but having hope, faith and belief that something bigger and better lies ahead is a relief. An example of this is when my sisters and I started a business together and were so adamant that it would be a success. We spoke about the big plans we had for our business and the financial growth we envisioned. When this did not come to fruition and we had to close down the business, we were distraught. I have now come to realise that God has bigger plans and I need to remain hopeful in that.

Finances are crucial to our day-to-day and allow us to enjoy what the world has to offer. This to me means being responsible with the way I handle my finances to enjoy these things in the healthiest way. It is also important so that I can be in a position to give willingly, generously and cheerfully. When my finances are taken care of, I can be in a better position to help others when needed.

On that note, this is the last chapter of my journey in the form of a business lifecycle. It has been a pleasure sharing my life journey with you to date – the journey continues. Thank you very much for taking your time to read through it. Life is a journey, and we are all in it together so let's be kind to one another and walk through this journey with one another knowing that God's got this! Life can throw so much at us, but just know that those times do not last forever (I have seen this with my own eyes).

Matthew 6:33 reads 'Seek first the kingdom of God and his righteousness, and all these things will be added onto you'. This verse to me means that partnering with God and allowing Him to work in our lives can reap so many rewards. As mentioned, to me this means working hard and allowing God to do the rest. Trusting God can provide tangible rewards, but most importantly the reward of constantly being content even when our plans fail, therefore having hope and faith that God always has something better in store. There may be seasons where we work hard, however our finances are not a true reflection of the hard work, and there are other seasons where this is visible. For those challenging seasons, I am learning to have faith and trust that God's timing is best. I have seen this countless times as God continues to bless me in various seasons of my life. For the seasons where things are looking dry, the faith I am developing has me believing that I will soon reap with the intention of blessing others generously too.

VULNERABILITY

Following on from my last chapters of my life journey in the form of a business lifecycle, I would like to take you through topics that have spoken volumes to me as I have written this book. The first topic is 'vulnerability'. Over the past few years, I have been seeing and experiencing the impacts of vulnerability. Sometimes, we feel as though we are going through life experiences alone. Through sharing, I have seen and experienced how the pain we hold onto can be released. Sharing can empower those around us to also share and release their pain or feel less alone. It takes a lot to be vulnerable, therefore definitely not something to be taken lightly. If you have read my previous chapters, you will begin to understand what it took for me to reach the stage of becoming more vulnerable.

In this chapter, I will be going through how various areas of my life are going to date as I am writing this. I will go through how I am working to push through and stay consistent – it isn't always easy, but fighting through those negative thoughts is key.

As mentioned at the start of this book, vulnerability in relationships is important. I have witnessed vulnerability strengthen my relationships, whether it be familial, romantic, or a friendship.

As mentioned in previous chapters, I struggled with having healthy boundaries in all my relationships. I am continuously working to create healthy boundaries in my relationships. I am not saying I have nailed it, but I am now aware that boundaries in a relationship need to be addressed based on how a particular situation is making me feel. I have learnt the power of saying no if I physically or mentally cannot meet a request. I have learnt that being open and honest helps solve so many unnecessary problems. I have seen the power of taking care of myself first because if I don't, then how can I possibly show up for others in the best possible way? I am definitely continuing with this approach because who doesn't want strong relationships, right?

In previous chapters, I took you through my career journey. In my career, I am continuing to learn as I face different challenges each day, but I am enjoying the growth journey. I am continuing with my lunchtime walks and taking breaks away from my desk. I am finding time to schedule my runs and also time to do the other things I enjoy – I have learnt that a balance is so important! Of course, there are busy seasons where 'life is just lifing', and it feels like the days are just whizzing by, but keeping on top of your health and self-care during those seasons is vital. Managing other areas of life without prioritising health can put us in constant survival mode – from experience, that's a 'NO' from me!

I am continuously working on being consistent with attending church to strengthen relationships at church and with God. I am continuing to read scripture, working on being more consistent. Spending time and connecting with God is such a beautiful thing. Prayer, reading the verse of the day in the mornings and ending the day with reading the Bible has been such a game-changer. Listening to God's voice to lead me wherever He calls me has put my mind at ease. No longer do I have to rely on doing things in my own strength, but with hard work and determination then leaving the rest to God, I am seeing amazing and beautiful things happen. I can definitely feel a change in myself for the better and I just smile to myself and say – it's all You, God.

As a member of the hosting/welcoming team at church, I received a text message from the hosting team leader one Sunday morning asking me if I was happy to share a message with the group about something God has spoken to me about. This was at the start of 2023. Years back, I would have declined for the fear of being vulnerable. Although I did not know what I would speak about, I sat down to think, and the blog I started in 2022 (which has formed this book) came to mind. This is what I shared with the group:

In 2022, I felt as though God was telling me to dig deep into all areas of my life and stay reminded of how far I have come. In 2022, I built the courage to start a blog where I wrote about the journey of all areas of my life to date; relationships, career, spirituality, health and finances. Through writing the blog, I could feel God's presence pouring into me as I shared. I knew this was the case because of all the wonderful comments I received about how my blog was inspiring readers and how relatable the things we don't often speak about were. This year, I feel as though God wants me to continue building on these areas with patience. This means being patient with myself when things are not happening at the pace I want them to, but doing all I can and leaving the rest to God. Through patience, I have seen wonderful things from God in various areas of my life – and I feel truly blessed. I will continue to channel patience knowing that God knows the plans He has for me, plans to prosper me and not to harm me, plans to give me a hope and a future as it is said in Jeremiah 29:11.

Vulnerability is such a powerful thing and allows us to connect with each other in the most beautiful way. It is not always easy to know how a person is feeling, why they behave the way they do, or why they make the decisions they make. It is not always for us to know but through opening up, it allows us to have more understanding, empathy and grace towards one another, which I definitely always appreciate.

2 Corinthians 6:11-13 reads 'We have spoken freely to you, Corinthians, and opened our hearts to you. We are not withholding our affection from you, but you are withholding yours from us. As a fair exchange – I speak as to my children – open wide your hearts'. This verse to me signifies the importance of vulnerability as Paul addresses the Corinthians. Through opening our hearts, we allow others to relate with us which can help others

feel less alone. It shows that we are working together and working as a community through the many ups and downs of life. Praying for each other and just being there for one another helps us build powerful bonds.

THE POWER OF MANIFESTATION

Another topic that has spoken volumes to me over the years is 'the power of manifestation' and my experience in relation to this topic to date.

In May 2023, I attended a powerful and inspiring five-day challenge called 'The Reinvent Yourself' challenge, hosted by a talented and inspiring self-discovery coach called Montelle Bee.[12] I received some really valuable lessons from the challenge. One of the tasks was to write down a crazy faith vision consisting of the vision you have for your life in the next 12 months. This was a challenge that encouraged me to overcome limiting beliefs by allowing faith to overcome fear. When I initially wrote down my crazy faith vision and shared it, I was definitely not thinking big enough, and there were elements of fear creeping in. After being encouraged to think bigger, I recreated my crazy faith vision and shared it with the group. As I wrote it, focusing on all areas of my life, I could really see myself living the dream life I had written. I was romanticising my life and having faith that I was capable of having this life I had written down. I began to smile, which gave me the push I needed to put all the steps in place to achieve this vision.

After the challenge, I then came across a sermon by Sarah Jakes Roberts titled 'Don't drop the call'.[14] This was so relatable after having completed the five-day challenge as detailed above. I felt goosebumps and knew that this was surely a sign from God. He is definitely working through me day in and day out, allowing me to stay true to my purpose by not letting fear or doubt overshadow the light within me. This also made me reflect upon the things in life that fuel me with passion, but somewhere along the line, I stop following through with that passion. Not because I have lost passion in that particular area, but because I have allowed fear or doubt to take over. It made me realise that to continue to stay connected with my passions, I need to stay reminded of the end goal. Staying connected to God and having fruitful communities are also really helpful in keeping me encouraged. Over time, I have developed some really fruitful communities through church, through fitness, and also through the challenge I took part in. The aim is to now stay connected and continue to remain encouraged on this amazing growth journey of mine.

When I was encouraged to think bigger during the challenge, it took me back to the times I placed certain limitations on myself. When I started to believe, have faith in the awesome human being God has created, and value myself, I then started thinking bigger. I thought about the things I have had faith in so far in the past few years, such as becoming a homeowner, which came to fruition. I manifested my dream career, which came to fruition. I manifested amazing communities and experiences that have also come to fruition. These things did not always come in the package I envisioned or planned for myself but all I can say is that God definitely came through with His bigger and better plan. It just required me to have faith!

As mentioned, I then created big visions for myself, which I prayed would come to fruition. I used the 12-week year plan to help me exercise the discipline I need. The five-day challenge included the provision of a 12-week year template[57] that helps track the daily steps you will be taking to achieve the set goals. I understand that manifestations may not always come in the way I want them to, but believe that if they do not, something better lies ahead. Watch this space and remember to dream and think big – work towards those goals step by step, in faith, and bask in abundance.

Matthew 21:22 reads 'Jesus replied, "Truly I tell you, if you have faith and do not doubt, not only can you do what was done to the fig tree, but also you can say to this mountain 'Go throw yourself into the sea', and it will be done. If you believe, you will receive whatever you ask for in prayer."'. This verse sums up how having faith, hope and belief is extremely important. It has helped me through some very challenging situations in which I could not see a way forward. As mentioned, although things may not always come in the way we imagined, the faith, the hope and the belief allow us to see beyond the disappointment and have allowed me to believe that there was a reason for it and better lies ahead. I have mentioned this multiple times throughout this book just to highlight how important this has been in all elements of my life. As a person who is always seeking for what's next and making plans for my future, this has been a powerful reminder when my plans have not always gone my way.

STAYING CONNECTED

In April 2023, I took a two-week holiday to my home country Malawi. What an awesome two weeks it was. Props to my sister for putting together a plan of activities for each stage of the trip (there was a lot of movement from one location to another throughout the trip, but it was definitely worth it!).

Our first destination was the capital, Lilongwe. From there, we drove five hours to Blantyre, another major city in Malawi to attend my cousin's wedding. The wedding was amazing, bringing family members from all over the country together. It also allowed me to see and connect with family members I had not seen in years. It was such a joyous event.

After the wedding, we stayed in Blantyre and visited a few places before making our way to Likoma Island on Lake Malawi, where my mother was brought up. The island is simply beautiful. When we arrived, my mother made many stops around the village, visiting family and friends. Everyone around the village was so friendly that everywhere we went, we would greet each and every individual along the way. Life there is so calm and peaceful. What most people do before they start their day is take a trip to the lake to bathe before heading home to proceed with their day-to-day activities. It took me a little while to adjust, but I gradually started to feel at home.

My mum, sister, and I then took a 45-minute boat trip across the lake from Likoma to Cobue (a small lake-side town in Niassa Province, in north-west Mozambique). The trip to Mozambique was a very special moment as I got to spend some much-needed time with my grandmother. As soon as we arrived, we were welcomed with open arms. My grandmother was extremely happy to see us. We conversed, sang, and danced with her, enjoying each and every moment. We were informed that all the Nkhalambas lived in the area – it was a pretty large area. As people passed my grandmother's house, they would greet us, and their relation to us was explained. I felt connected to my roots in that moment, feeling proud of my Nkhalamba name, and felt right at home. When it was time to leave, I felt emotional, but at the same time, I was so grateful for the time I had spent with my grandmother and my relatives from my father's side.

We then headed back to Likoma to prepare for our journey back to the mainland. The next phase of the trip included sightseeing and some relaxation at a gorgeous lodge. It gave me time to reflect and really appreciate my beautiful beloved country.

When it was time to head back to the UK, I felt many mixed emotions. As a person who remains sane by having a routine, I was eager to get back to my routine after two weeks out of it. At the same time, I was not ready to leave behind the beautiful memories I had created. I am still looking back at photos and videos to this day, smiling back to myself.

This trip has taught me that creating and maintaining family connections is very important. As much as we try to run away from it, life is short and fragile. I am learning to treasure each moment, nourish fruitful connections, and remember just how precious life is. Moving forward, my intention is to make time to spend with loved ones.

When I got back from my trip, the first back to church service I attended was powerful! The pastor preached about how we tend to spend most of our time working and fail to intentionally prepare time for rest. We work until we burn out, and when our bodies cry out for rest, our immediate response would probably be to sit on the sofa, watch Netflix, and endlessly scroll through social media. This resonated with me, and it made me realise that I had to change up my routine. This means doing as much work as I physically can throughout the week (avoiding burnout) to intentionally prepare and make room for rest at the weekends (aiming to fit in work, errands and chores during the week – by prioritising and fitting in the things I can, leaving the weekends for leisure). Leisure to me looks like self-care by checking in with myself and spending some quality time with family and friends. As we carry on with our day-to-day activities, let's take some time to think about the things that truly matter in life and intentionally make room for them. Building memories with those we love is so valuable in this life.

Genesis 2:18 reads 'The Lord God said 'It is not good for the man to be alone. I will make a helper suitable for him'. Having community is a vital element of the human experience. Without community, we cannot get very far in life. Although I believe that God is our ultimate helper, this verse clarifies how God has put others on earth to help us through Him. A helper in this verse goes beyond a life partner, but everyone who is around and gives us encouragement through the ups and down of life. This varies from friends, family and anyone else we are in connection with. Connection in this day and age comes in various forms. I enjoy watching YouTube vlogs of people that I find inspiring and people whose lives I can relate to. The aim for some of the vloggers I watch is to create a community through their vlogs by sharing relatable content and allowing subscribers to like or comment on their content. Although virtual, this is another form of connection.

As mentioned before, this verse goes beyond a life partner being the helper. Growing up, I always equated this verse to marriage and felt disconnected from it when marriage was not coming my way. As I have begun to cultivate more relationships through family, friendships and communities this verse now speaks volumes. Staying connected with all the people that add value to my life as I add value to theirs has made me realise that I am not alone and has made this verse very relatable. I have a multitude of suitable helpers that God has blessed me with, and I am grateful for that. Staying connected with them is necessary to ensure I am giving back what God has given me through offering my service and gifts to others.

THE VALUE OF COMMUNITY

In different chapters of this book, I have referenced how having a community is so valuable. I understand that God did not create us all in this world to purely live in isolation. There are times when isolation is necessary (which will be explored in the next chapter), but primarily community is something to be cherished. Outside of friendships, it has taken me time to be a part of meaningful communities. As stated in many parts of this book, age 30 was a real game-changer in my life. At 30, I decided to go on my first ever fitness holiday (mentioned later in this book) which was advertised by a fitness community that I had joined. I was initially nervous about signing up for it as at this time I did not know members of the community well. I talked myself out of the fears and procrastination of booking the holiday and proceeded to do it anyway. I contacted the host of the fitness holiday Despina[15] and booked myself in.

The fitness holiday experience is explained later in this book. I built meaningful friendships and learnt so much about myself on the trip. It was truly unexpected. I then started attending the events the community would host and enjoyed connecting with people at different stages of life as well as backgrounds. I connected with people from different walks of life who have now become friends. People who have really pushed me and challenged me beyond my limits and have helped me reignite the power inside of me. People who I would not have met due to not being in the same circles, but have had the opportunity to meet due to meeting them during the holiday and at the hosted events. I am so grateful to this day for the hand that God has had in giving me the courage to book the holiday and get connected.

Building communities within church has also given me so much joy. In my earlier years of church-hopping, which then resulted in tuning into church online, I often found it hard to believe that I would get to a place of having a church family. Hillsong church is the first church that created this atmosphere for me. Being a part of the church made me want to get involved in being a part of the welcome team. Being a part of the church welcome team involves getting to church earlier to make sure that the church foyer looks presentable before the service starts, welcoming people into the church, making sure people feel comfortable by finding them seats in church and ensuring that people feel genuinely welcome. Being a part of the team helped me connect with other team members as well as church attendees coming into church, therefore building meaningful relationships with them. The welcome team community has really helped me grow in faith. Team members have really encouraged me by seeing the value that I bring to the team. There are times that I have failed to see the good qualities that God has placed inside of me and most of the time, having the right communities can help and encourage you to see these qualities. I have realised that being able to see these qualities as well as praying about these, can help lead you to finding your calling and God-given purpose. I have seen this in my life and the day I realised this, I received true joy.

From being a welcome team member, I then started to look into other teams at church that I wanted to be involved in. I had an interest in being part of the sisterhood team and from this I started attending the sisterhood connect group. This provided me with a community of sisters in church who were going through various challenges and joys in life (open enough to share their stories) and how God is working in their lives. Being a part of this community gave me true joy. As mentioned at the start of this book, life is not a journey we should look to embark on on our own. Having a community of people who motivate and inspire you is such a relief. The sisterhood community at church has ladies from different backgrounds, different ages and women at different stages of life. I have gained so much wisdom from the ladies which has helped me and is continuing to help me grow in my faith.

Community has played such a big role in my life. I have seen the importance of being in a community of people who make you feel comfortable opening up, people who energise you and people who lift your spirit. I have found that some of my low days have turned into energised days after spending time with the communities that I have built up which gives me reassurance that they are the right communities.

Proverbs 27:17 reads 'As iron sharpens iron, so one person sharpens another'. From this verse I understand that finding the right communities of people who can speak life into you, challenge you to become a better version of yourself and encourage you on the days you do not have the courage is of vital importance. In turn being that for others within your community are ingredients for a fruitful community. As said before, the communities that I have mentioned above have done that for me. In the chapters above, I have mentioned the tools and resources I have used to work on myself so that I can aim to be the best version of myself each day. I understand that doing the work within ourselves can help us attract the communities that are good for us and that help us to grow in the best way. This in turn helps us also pour into the communities we are part of.

ISOLATION

Although there are seasons for staying fully connected with people, I have also come to understand the power of isolation at various points in life. I realised that isolation can be a powerful tool in my 30s. Before this, I saw isolation as such a terrible thing and always associated this with being a 'loner'. When isolation comes in intervals, I have come to appreciate that it is sometimes needed when done intentionally. During my seasons of intentional isolation, I made sure that I was fully prepared before entering the season. Preparation to me is making sure I am aware of the goals and things that I would like to work on during the season. Preparation also looks like ensuring that I have freed up my calendar to focus on these things without distractions, but also ensuring that I am available for my community when absolutely necessary. This means creating boundaries with my community before going into isolation by informing them of the things I can and cannot be available for in that particular season, therefore creating an understanding.

During my intentional seasons of isolation, I have found so much power in connecting with God and being present, therefore allowing Him to guide my steps. I have seen many miraculous things happen by doing this, which has definitely strengthened my relationship with

God. During these seasons, many beautiful ideas that link into various aspects of my life have come together and this has been such an amazing thing to see. During these seasons I also learn so many things about myself which is always useful before going back into the world where so many opinions exist. This has helped me stay grounded in seasons of doubt, worry and fear because the more I do it, the more I begin to understand myself and what I truly stand for.

Seasons of isolation can also be referred to as wilderness seasons in biblical terms.[56] In the Bible we see people like Moses, the Israelites, David and Jesus go through wilderness seasons. Wilderness seasons can often be challenging, and we see that even Jesus faced challenging times during His wilderness season. The great thing about going into a wilderness season is that I am silencing all the noises of the world and keeping my focus on God's word so that I can clearly hear Him. There have been many times where I could feel the weight of the world coming down on me in terms of my career, relationships and health as mentioned in earlier chapters of this book. In these times I felt so far away from God because I had allowed the opinions of the world to cloud my judgment. The times when I have gone into isolation to connect with God have allowed me to truly hear what He is saying to me. Whether it is to continue waiting for the right relationships for me, continue waiting for the job opportunity that gives me a spark or to continue having the strength I need and the strength He gives me to get through some daily challenges. Moments of isolation can also bring about temptation. There have been times I have felt that God telling me to wait for certain things was taking too long which created the temptation for me to do things in my own will – time and time again this has not been beneficial.

I have come to find that seasons of isolation/wilderness seasons are to be cherished and to be done intentionally with a plan before going into them. I definitely plan to have many more of these. Although life may often seem too busy to go into a wilderness season, a wilderness season is definitely the best thing to help manage the busyness of life. Spending time with God definitely teaches me to focus on the things that truly matter.

Acts 7:38 reads 'He was in the assembly in the wilderness, with the angel who spoke to him on Mount Sinai and with our ancestors; and he received living words to pass on to us'. This verse of Moses going into the wilderness and receiving the living words to pass on allows me to understand that going into a wilderness season means being fully connected with God in that moment of isolation to hear Him clearly so that when I go back into the busy, chaotic world, I can go out and spread the good news that He has given me. It clarifies that this season is temporary because as mentioned at the start there are seasons to be fully connected with people which is a season that requires intentionality too. Going into a wilderness season should be understood as a season of receiving God's wonderful gifts to then pass them onto others in the seasons of connection.

IMPOSTER SYNDROME

In an earlier chapter, 'Career Survival', I touched upon imposter syndrome, described as 'the persistent inability to believe that one's success is deserved or has been legitimately achieved as a result of one's own efforts or skills'.[2] Throughout my career and life, I am realising how imposter syndrome often creeps up no matter how much I try to get rid of it. I feel as though once I have achieved a successful outcome in life, the feeling of success does not last long and I quickly ponder upon the next things or the many other things I have not achieved. I have tried so hard to change my mindset when it comes to imposter syndrome.

In August 2023, I stumbled across a podcast by a coach called Caroline Flanagan.[13] Who spoke about making imposter syndrome your strength. This is the first time I had heard anyone speak about making imposter syndrome a strength.

I listened to an episode of the podcast which spoke about making imposter syndrome your strength and gained some valuable lessons that I will be taking going forward.[58] In this podcast the coach spoke about making imposter syndrome a strength rather than a weakness and highlights that imposter syndrome is not a problem you should try to fix. It should act as a reminder that you are extraordinary and unique and have taken an unconventional path to be here. This hit me hard because as a black African woman, I grew up in a culture where speaking up for myself as a child was generally considered rude. As a woman who is now required to speak up for myself in all areas of my life, breaking this chain has been and is still oftentimes a long process. This feeds into my imposter syndrome. When I heard the coach speak about how imposter syndrome is a reminder of this it hit home. She speaks about leaning into your imposter syndrome and not allowing it to hold you back, but allowing it to distinguish you so that you learn to use it to your advantage. Knowing your value and celebrating your imposter syndrome should therefore allow you to stop over-working and over-thinking but instead allow you to focus on how your unconventional path can bring value to everything you do.

I also sometimes battle with feelings of not being good enough no matter how hard I try. This often leads to me feeling stressed and anxious, therefore leading me to comparing myself to others. Being a woman of faith allows me to lean more into this and realise that although I may feel successful in some seasons and less successful in other seasons, the core of my success lies in knowing that God has got me and no matter the negative opinions I place on myself or others place on me. I should always remember that I am fearfully and wonderfully made. Oftentimes, when I start to feel anxious, I speak to myself out loud reminding myself that 'I am fearfully and wonderfully made', therefore I have no reason to ever think that I am not good enough. The thoughts creep in but it is my responsibility to make that conscious and intentional effort to snap out of it. Life changes and there are various seasons where we may feel that all is working out according to ours and God's plans and there are seasons where we may feel lost, confused with feelings of inadequacy. If this is you, I challenge you from today to start combatting any of those negative thoughts about yourself and be more intentional about replacing those thoughts with positive ones. You are amazing and I believe that all of us are fearfully and wonderfully made with so much to bring into this world. So, whether it is being a supportive family member, a supportive friend or someone who brings light and hope to your community – you are a blessing to this world. We should be more intentional about bringing out the gifts that are within us. Being good enough should not be linked to our status or career as these things change and when they do they can leave us doubting ourselves. I therefore challenge you to dig deep and find the gifts within you and place value in that.

I have created the below affirmations to affirm me when those imposter syndrome thoughts creep in. They affirm me knowing that my true strength lies in God and I am His vessel bringing His work to life:

- I am resourceful through God
- I am disciplined through God
- I am dedicated through God
- I work hard through God
- I am confident through God
- I am a leader through God

Psalms 139:14 reads 'I praise you because I am fearfully and wonderfully made; your works are wonderful, I know that full well'. No matter the amount of times that imposter syndrome forces its way in my life, staying rooted in this verse is the best reminder that I am extremely valuable and I do not have to spend my time proving this to anyone other than myself and God. Time spent doing this is definitely wasted time and energy that becomes draining. I have learnt to always do my best in everything I do, but pushing above and beyond to prove my worth to others is definitely not worth it or fulfilling in the long run.

SINGLE SEASON

As mentioned in previous chapters, my goal and plan for life was to be married by the age of 25 and when this did not happen, I was disappointed. When I reached 30 and this had still not happened, I began to understand that this was okay, and I was whole even without a husband. I realised that I had allowed the opinions of others and of society to have so much influence on me which led me into thinking that I needed a husband to be whole. Reaching 30 was definitely the golden age for me as I felt that I was really beginning to understand and value myself a lot more than I had previously. As mentioned in previous chapters there are various tools that helped me to achieve this level of self-worth, as well as a growth in my relationship with God.

I realised that my single season was a season to truly connect with myself and figure out who I am before a husband came into the picture. My 30s is when I started doing activities that I enjoy unapologetically, which are mentioned in my previous chapters. Doing these activities and connecting with various people through these activities has brought me true joy. Being 'single' should not be associated with 'shame' or 'being a loner', but it should rather be embraced. There are so many experiences in this life that can be done without having a husband. Finding the joy from these experiences has taught me to be happy on my own so that when the 'one' does come along, it is a bonus.

Throughout my single season I have experienced so many blessings and opportunities from God that are building my character. Connecting with God has been an essential part of my single season. My relationship with God has had its ups and downs and I am now at a stage where I feel my relationship is much stronger compared to where it was. I now know that God knows what I need in the various seasons of my life. Reaching 30 and being in a single season has definitely had its challenges, but by having God by my side I have seen the many blessings of this season.

Ecclesiastes 3:1-8: 'There is a time for everything, and a season for every activity under the heavens: 2 – a time to be born and a time to die, a time to plant and a time to uproot, 3 – a time to kill and a time to heal, a time to tear down and a time to build, 4 – a time to weep and a time to laugh, a time to mourn and a time to dance, 5 – a time to scatter stones and a time to gather them, a time to embrace and a time to refrain from embracing, 6 – a time to search and a time to give up, a time to keep and a time to throw away, 7 – a time to tear and a time to mend, a time to be silent and a time to speak, 8 – a time to love and a time to hate, a time for war and a time for peace.' God has seasons for everything and I believe He is working in us to prepare us for each season we are about to enter. It often feels like God has forgotten about us in those preparation seasons but I have come to learn that He is with us every step of the way.

PREPARING FOR MARRIAGE

Marriage is something that has always been on my heart since I was a young girl. In the earlier chapters, I touched on this and how I had thought '25' is the age I would be married. To me, marriage marked completeness and for years I believed that marriage made me whole. I thought that without marriage something was definitely wrong with me. When I passed the age of 25 without marriage, I began to grow weary. It was in my 30s that I realised that marriage did not complete me and that I was whole on my own as explained above. I realised that God had created me as a whole person with so much more to give to this world. My 30s is when I truly began to explore the things that I liked and disliked as well as the things that gave me purpose and passion. In earlier chapters I explained the tools and resources that I used to really dig deep and truly discover myself. When I was younger, I spoke about how I thought love is all I needed to make a marriage work, but I discovered in my 30s that there was so much more. I look back at my past relationships and begin to understand the reason they did not work and that God had been leading me into a different direction.

In my 30s I became intentional about my single season as explained in the chapter above. I began to understand that isolation is a time for preparation and if we are obedient to God's voice in this time, God can speak words of wisdom and guide us to where He is calling us. This involves prayer, reading the word and using that time to focus on Him. At the age of 33, there was a lot that I had learnt about relationships and that the journey is challenging but with God by my side, I do not have to carry the burdens and challenges alone. I am still learning about relationships and marriage and have come to the realisation that marriage is still a journey and is not the end of the love story. I have come to realise that marriage is beautiful in that it has its challenges but the beauty is seen in how two people come together and navigate those challenges. Navigating the challenges means understanding that love is not only a feeling but a choice and that keeping God at the centre of a relationship allows the relationship to thrive. I am still on the journey of learning and discovering more about relationships and marriages and that journey continues.

1 Corinthians 13:4-8 reads 'Love is patient, love is kind... Love never fails'. From this verse I understand that love is truly more a choice than a feeling as mentioned above. If this is done with reciprocity by both parties, I have come to understand how beautiful love can be. A choice to be patient with the other person and to understand their point of view rather than rushing into assumptions. A choice to be kind to the other person, even during difficult times. Then when love is made a choice with God at the centre of it all, it is more likely to lead to a successful marriage.

SELF-CARE VS. SOUL CARE

Self-care and soul-care are both very important and I believe that they should always be prioritised. When we look after ourselves and our needs, we can then have the capacity to care for those around us. Self-care is described as the practice of taking care of your physical and mental health which promotes your overall wellbeing.[7] Soul-care, on the other hand, is the daily process of nurturing and renewing your soul under the guidance of the Holy Spirit.[8]

I have found that when I fail to prioritise self-care and soul-care, I start going into survival mode as described in my previous chapters. As said in previous chapters, survival mode is never a good place to be. Discovering and practicing soul-care and self-care has really changed my life for the better. Towards the end of this book is my 'Self-Care Toolkit' which I use when I start to feel my mood becoming low. All of these things have helped to pick me up when I am having 'one of those days'. This, along with soul-care – prayer, devotion and quality time with God – have served me well until this day! I urge you today to discover your 'Self-Care Toolkit' as well as your soul-care to truly thrive and cater to your needs so that you can continue being your best version for yourself as well as those around you!

1 Corinthians 6:19-20 reads 'Do you not know that your bodies are of the Holy Spirit who is in you, whom you

have received from God? You are not your own; you were bought at a price. Therefore honour God with your bodies'. This to me emphasises how God wants us to practice self-care by honouring and looking after our physical and mental bodies. This to me means feeding our bodies and minds with things that will nourish us and set us up to be the best versions of ourselves.

Matthew 11:28 reads 'Come to me, all you who are weary and burdened, and I will give you rest'. In this verse I believe God is calling us to practice soul-care. When we practice soul care, we renew our souls by being in God's presence and surrendering all our worries, fears and burdens unto Him. Soul-care has been a literal Godsend. There are many moments where things that I had planned had not gone my way and I had lost control. Knowing that I can surrender my plans to God so that He can take the wheel has been a heavy weight lifted off of my shoulders. This has definitely been the key to soul-care for me.

BOUNDARIES

Throughout the chapters of this book, it is evident that boundaries is an area that I severely struggled with in various aspects of my life including relationships and careers. It has been a journey and a journey that I am still on. Establishing and being clear of my boundaries has given me the space to truly discover myself and most importantly space to really reflect and develop my relationship with God. As mentioned in earlier chapters, we must get to the space of putting on our oxygen masks first so that we are in a better place to help others when we have the space to do so.

Being a people pleaser, I had little to no boundaries, often saying yes to things I did not have the capacity to do. This led to burnout and frustration. It is something that I still catch myself doing in my 30s but I am now more self-aware and examine the situation before I say yes. Being burnt out can make us realise that we need to put boundaries in place when it becomes too late, which I have experienced multiple times.

I have realised that boundaries need to be exercised in all areas of life to allow this to become a habit. I have noticed that when I do not exercise boundaries in my career/work life, for example, this feeds into me not exercising boundaries in my relationships for example.

However, when boundaries are exercised in all areas of my life, I have seen myself thriving. I have also noticed that this allows me to prioritise my soul-care as well as self-care as mentioned in the previous chapter. The balance is not always easy but so worth it. In moments where I feel that my boundaries have gone out of the window and have therefore fed into all areas of my life, I know it is a time I need to really connect with God as well as seek therapy. Knowing when I am getting to this point and seeking the necessary help has known to serve me well. Journaling has also helped me to keep track of my thoughts and make note of the patterns. Getting to a point where I feel myself thriving because I am respecting my boundaries gives me the drive to get back to this place when boundaries have gone out of the window. Surely that is motivation enough and I can honestly tell you it definitely is!

Proverbs 4:23 reads 'Above all else, guard your heart, for everything you do flows from it'. This verse to me emphasises that once we set boundaries with those around us, this allows us to look after ourselves so that we can have a full cup to then release good energy. As mentioned, when I respect my boundaries, I feel myself thriving and prioritising self-care and soul-care which brings abundance to my life. So, as the verse says, look after yourself and your heart then good things will definitely flow from that!

SELF-DISCIPLINE & CONSISTENCY

Self-discipline is the ability to control your actions and behaviour to achieve a goal or maintain a standard of conduct.[53] Consistency, on the other hand, is the quality of always behaving or performing in a similar way.[54]

Throughout my life I have seen how consistency over time leads to self-discipline. This has been true in all areas of my life so far. When I am consistent in ensuring I prioritise my time with God (getting into the word, listening to worship music, devotional time, etc.) I have noticed that, over time, my relationship with God has definitely become stronger and it makes it natural to seek God in all areas of my life.

When I am consistent in maintaining my relationships, I have noticed that it becomes natural for me to schedule quality time with those around me to truly connect. Therefore, in this way consistency has led to self-discipline as I know that the continuous maintenance of relationships requires me pouring into my relationships as I receive from those relationships.

When I am consistent with progressing in my career, I have noticed that it has become natural for me to say yes to the opportunities that align with my goals. This means having the self-discipline of saying yes to the right opportunities and working hard to make those opportunities a success. As I say yes to the right opportunities, it has also given me the self-discipline to explore the opportunities further to see what other opportunities that could lead to. For example, saying yes to an opportunity at work to go to a women's conference and then present how the day went to my team as well as write an article has led to me being recognised in the company. This opportunity also opened up my eyes to other opportunities such as becoming chartered in my career and taking the necessary steps to do so.

When I am consistent in my finances, I have noticed that it then becomes natural for me to really think of the purchases I am making before I make them. This has helped me build the self-discipline to manage my finances better, which makes a huge difference.

When I am consistent in prioritising my mental and physical health, I have noticed that consistency over time has led me to have the self-discipline to crave for healthier options which requires taking the necessary actions to put healthy habits in place. For my physical health an example of this looks like getting in the habit of working out at least three times a week (there are times I fall off, but the self-discipline has made it easy for me to get back on my feet when I do). For my mental health, an example of this looks like having my go-to self-care and soul-care toolkits and putting them in place as habits to incorporate into my life.

Luke 8:15 reads 'But the seed on good soil stands for those with a noble and good heart, who hear the word, retain it, and by persevering produce crop'. This verse speaks volumes and captures the benefits of consistency. I have noticed that perseverance and consistency definitely reap rewards which bring joy. Through consistency and perseverance, self-discipline is developed which allows for an abundance of rewards.

MY HACKS

I have included some topics that you may find of interest in relation to health and fitness. These are topics that have also really helped me along my journey and include some things that I have done to date.

HEALTH AND FITNESS

A hack to managing the to-do lists of life

Sometimes life can become overwhelming when you have so many goals, so much on your to-do list and life is just 'lifing'. An amazing method that I have started using to plan life out and ensure that things get done is the 12-week year.[3] To find out more about the 12-week year, find the book here: https://www.amazon.co.uk/12-Week-Year-Others-Months/dp/1118509234. This has helped me manage stress when I am feeling overwhelmed with my goals and to do list – it provides a structured and visually clear way to organising my goals.

This has helped to keep me mentally sane through the goals and responsibilities of life, ensuring that I am proactive in hitting my goals. Having a weekly plan to help achieve your goals in small chunks makes it seem so much easier, simpler and smoother to achieve those goals.

My favourite 'made up' go-to green smoothie:

Below are the ingredients to my 'go-to' green smoothie. This smoothie provides me with the energy I need to start my day and also ensures I get a portion of greens in the most delicious way. This smoothie is sweet with a little tang added from the ginger. I normally take this smoothie in the morning along with my vitamins for that morning energy boost:

- A handful of spinach
- 1 medium Apple
- 1 medium pear
- A medium glass of apple juice
- An inch piece of raw ginger
- Half a cucumber

Self-Care Toolkit:

When I am having one of those days and my mood is low, these are the things I like to do to pick me up:

1. Prayer, reading my Bible, and listening to gospel music often give me the pick-up I need (in general connecting with God)
2. Listen to or create your own affirmations – say them out loud as I look into the mirror, repeat them twice and really believe in them (positive things only because I am a fearfully and wonderfully made gem – so are you!)
3. Listen to music and dance to wherever the beat takes me

4. Dressing up and going out on a solo date – this can consist of anything you enjoy. I enjoy a meal and then the cinema
5. Getting some body products and pampering myself at home (face mask, nail kit, etc.)
6. Doing exercise that I enjoy (I enjoy running and dancing which often give me the boost and energy I need)
7. Making myself a healthy treat – I enjoy making smoothies which I find fun to make and delicious to snack on giving me that 'feel good' feeling

Running tips:[4]

I started running during the 2020 lockdown and since then it has become part of my lifestyle, and I love it. I have picked up tips along the way which make it an enjoyable activity – here they are:

1. Get good and comfortable running shoes. I bought myself a pair of running shoes which connect to a running app. They coach me as I run, helping me with my body form as well as pace.
2. Stretch, stretch and stretch – do not underestimate the power of a good stretch after a run. Stretching for about 15 minutes can ensure that the knees are getting a good stretch to avoid knee injuries.

    A good knee stretch video can be found here: https://www.youtube.com/watch?v=LsB2mEMA1wk

A good beginner full body stretch:[5] https://www.youtube.com/watch?v=-SD_MucCa6c

3. Get yourself some knee guards to support those knees as you run.
4. Breathing in and out whilst running helps avoid running out of breath.
5. Creating a running playlist to motivational music can help provide that confidence boost
6. A consistent amount of runs per week (for example at least three times a week (5k runs)) can help with building up momentum

FITNESS HOLIDAY

You may be wondering what a fitness holiday entails.[15] I had the exact same question! I have so far attended two fitness holidays – first one to Cyprus in September 2022 and second one to Croatia in May 2024. All I can say is that it was an amazing experience mixing fitness with holiday elements such as sightseeing and exploration. Below is the timetable of my revival fitness holiday to Cyprus, detailing what I got up to.

What an amazing experience indeed! I met wonderful people (a community full of encouraging and positive individuals), I challenged myself both mentally and physically and succeeded. I definitely enjoyed many gorgeous views. I look forward to many more trips like this. Definitely value for money – peaceful, gorgeous accommodation with fun-packed activities as shown below. There are many more fitness holidays that I would like to attend in the future to have this amazing experience again. Below is the timetable of the first fitness holiday I attended.

Day 1:

09:25-09.55am: Bootcamp on the beach

10:05-10:45am: Pilates, Mobility, Core, Stretch

11:00-11:45am: Cubatone

17:00-18:00pm: Gentle Yoga Flow & Relaxation

Day 2 (Friday 16/09/2022):

05:30am-Midday: Akamas 7.5km Hike & Swim

16:00-19:30pm: Sunset Cruise (Adventure)

Day 3 (Saturday 17/09/2022):

09:00-09:45am: Pilates/Yoga Combo Prep

09:50-10:35am: Cubatone

10:40-11:25am: Poundfit

13:00-18:00pm: Buggy Trip (Adventure)

Day 4 (Sunday 18/09/2022):

09:10-09:55am: Gentle Yoga Flow

10:00-11:00am: Kangoo Boots

10:10-10:50am: Pilates core & stretch

11:05 am-12:05pm: Aqua Zumba/Freestyle

14:00pm: Limassol Exploration Trip

Day 5 (Monday 19/09/2022):

08:30am onwards: Massage therapies and departure

Having a community with similar interests to you is so beautiful and I have experienced the beauty in that with this fitness community. It gives me a chance to connect with people at different stages in life as well as from various backgrounds. It also allows me to enjoy elements of fun, exercise, holiday and food.

HALF-MARATHON

My First Half-Marathon Experience

I made the decision to sign up for my first half-marathon and completed this on 16/10/2022. As mentioned under the 'Healthy Tips' section of this book, under 'Running Tips', I started running during the 2022 lockdown and really enjoyed it. I used these running tips to assist me with my training for the half-marathon.

I aimed to complete the half-marathon in two hours but achieved this in two hours, 24 minutes. At first, I was gutted but I reflected and thought, *Woah, what an achievement!* It's funny what the mind can push the body to do.

As soon as I started the half-marathon, I filled my mind with the most positive thoughts. I kept telling myself, *You can do it, you got this, just keep going!* I was raising money for a charity that meant something to me, giving me the motivation I needed to keep going. A quarter way through, I thought to myself, *Three more quarters to go... keep going*, and so I did. There were points in time where it became so repetitive that my mind went blank but still I kept going. Anytime I needed a boost I would put my mind to work again telling it to push my little legs.

As soon as I reached 12 miles, my legs and feet were in so much pain... the last mile was the hardest for sure! It felt like it went on forever! As soon as I saw the finish line, I sprinted to the end. Once I crossed the finish line I was so proud of myself. I had finally done it – 13 miles! All the months of preparation had definitely paid off! All I can say is consistency is key! Stay consistent with the training, stay consistent with the positive mindset and the world is your oyster!

Then book yourself a nice massage/spa day afterwards... because you deserve it!

I went and got it done! It was an amazing challenge and achievement.

I completed another half-marathon in October 2024 and plan on doing many more – this allows me a chance to combine running (which I am now very fond of) and raising money for charities that are close to my heart. A full marathon? Maybe? Watch this space!

FASHION

Sustainable Fashion

On one of our walks, my sister and I spoke about the amount of clothes we have in our wardrobes and no longer wear. We also spoke about how there needs to be a better way of getting rid of unwanted clothes. I have slowly been transitioning my wardrobe, and it occurred to me that I am no longer interested in buying so many things! The amount of clothes I accumulated in the past was ridiculous – definitely quantity over quality (hoarder mentality!). In 2022, I decided to clear out my wardrobe, getting rid of all my 'washed out' poor quality clothing, and I am slowly starting to look into and invest in clothing that is of a higher quality. I am also starting to develop a more minimalistic attitude to clothing, therefore slowly purchasing items that will allow me to create my ideal capsule wardrobe. Starting a capsule wardrobe has made me realise how much easier it is to put an outfit together. I do a check of my wardrobe from time to time to remind myself of the clothes I have to stop me unnecessarily buying a similar piece of clothing.

I am also starting to feel more conscious about the impact that fast fashion has on the environment and how unsustainable this is. I am slowly taking steps to ensure my approach to fashion is more sustainable. As well as aiming to purchase high-quality clothing that will last longer, I have also opened a Vinted account[18] to sell clothing that is still in good condition, but I no longer wear.

As someone who enjoys shopping, I will continue to enjoy it whilst asking myself these questions before I make a purchase:[55]

1. Is the piece of clothing of good quality and will I be able to get over 30 wears from it?
2. Is the piece of clothing I want available in a store that promotes sustainable clothing? There are some good quality clothes on Vinted, therefore second-hand purchases are also a good way to go.
4. How many outfits can I create with a particular piece of clothing?
5. Do I really want the item in my wardrobe, and would I feel confident wearing it from time to time?

CONCLUSION

Thank you for reading through my life journey to date as well as topics that have had some true meaning throughout my journey. As mentioned, the journey continues as I learn more and explore more. I hope that this book offers some encouragement to someone reading. There are seasons of life that can test us and challenge us and there are also other seasons where life is moving in a direction that makes us feel content.

Through this book, I have gone through some of the methods and tools I have used to anchor me as I continue on this journey. The main thing I want you to take away is that God is faithful if you allow Him to work in your life. Hoping and trusting in Him through the good and bad times has allowed me to live a life of peace and hope no matter the season. When disappointing situations occur, I have learnt that it is okay to feel sad, angry and upset so long as we do not prolong these feelings, but get back up knowing that there is hope.

God has also blessed us with so many other people in the world who are experiencing life just as we are. There are so many people in this world that we can connect with based on common interests and genuine love and care for one another. I encourage you to find connections that fulfil you and make you feel like you are not alone. Love to you all – let's do this thing called life together! 'As individuals we are strong. Together, with God, we are unstoppable' – Rosemary M. Wixom[6]

Relationships – this journey started off rocky but through all the tools, resources and through God's hand in it all, I am at a place where I am managing my relationships much better. As I pour into others, I am allowing for others to pour into me. Relationships can come with many challenges and I am at a place where I can better manage the challenges that occur. I have learnt that communication and listening to understand can resolve a lot of problems in relationships. I also understand that needing to have difficult conversations should not be seen as a bad thing but something that strengthens relationships.

Career – this journey also started off rocky. I started off with so many doubts and insecurities and although I still have them now, they are not as severe as they initially were. Again, my relationship with God and the tools and resources He has provided me with give me the confidence and reassurance that I am fearfully and wonderfully made in Him. This provides me with all I need to keep on pushing and leaving anything out of my control to Him. This has helped me with the many opportunities that God has given me access to.

Spirituality – I have seen my growth in this journey in that my responses to situations have changed because of the decision I have made to put God first in all the situations in my life. Putting God first in all areas of my life has given me an unexplainable peace and joy. It is a journey I am still on as I continue to seek God and trust Him in all that He is doing in my life. It requires me to be obedient and listen for His voice in all that I do.

Health (physical and mental) – this journey also started rocky but I am now at a place where I realise that feeding my body and mind with the things that nourish it gives me the mental and physical capacity I need to achieve the goals I set myself. I have seen that this with God's guidance has been a real game-changer in my life. In terms of physical health, I have studied my body and know the foods that give me energy and the foods that drain my energy. I therefore look to avoid the energy draining foods as much as I can but still treat myself here and there. With physical health, I have seen how exercising in the mornings gives me the energy boost I need for the day. With my mental health, I have come to know what my triggers are and look to avoid certain situations that drain my energy.

Finances – this journey also started rocky but I now understand the importance of budgeting. Budgeting allows me to see where my money is going and to monitor the expenses that are my personal wants and needs. Involving God in my finances has also been very important.

As I conclude, I would like you to join me in examining and analysing all areas of your life as categorised in this book. Which areas are you looking to grow further in and what tools and resourcing are you using/would you like to use to help you achieve that growth? I believe that we all have the potential to be who God has called us to be. That can come with its challenges, but those challenges are all part of the resilience building.

ACKNOWLEDGEMENTS

I would like to say a special THANK YOU to all the people that have gone on this life journey with me.

I would first and foremost like to thank God for always being with me through every season even in the seasons that I felt He was distant. I look back at the difficult seasons in life which were really hard and my faith was low, but God really kept me going.

Secondly, I would like to thank you, Mum and Dad, for your unwavering support through every season of my life. From the sacrifices that you have made to allow me access to opportunities that have helped me in many areas of my life, to your constant love for me. You are truly a blessing.

I would also like to thank my siblings (Esther, Anastasia and John) for experiencing childhood with me. Thank you for being the ones that I can turn to through life's challenges as well as through the joys of life. We all have different versions and experiences of our childhood but the laughter that comes out of the memories we share gives me joy.

I also want to thank my family, friends, communities and mentors. Thank you for your wise words. Thank you for being there for me through life's storms and for also being there on the sunny days. Thank you for celebrating achievements and milestones with me. I am truly grateful.

REFERENCES

1. Cognitive Behaviour Therapy (CBT), accessed August 28, 2025, https://www.nhs.uk/mental-health/talking-therapies-medicine-treatments/talking-therapies-and-counselling/cognitive-behavioural-therapy-cbt/
2. Oxford English Dictionary, 'Imposter Syndrome', accessed August 28, 2025, https://www.oed.com/dictionary/impostor-syndrome_n?tl=true
3. 12 Week Year, accessed August 28, 2025, https://www.amazon.co.uk/12-Week-Year-Others-Months/dp/1118509234
4. Knee Pain Relief Stretches – 5 Minute Real Time Routine, accessed August 28, 2025, https://www.youtube.com/watch?v=LsB2mEMA1wk
5. 13 min. Full Body Stretch Routine For Tight Muscles| Beginner Friendly, accessed August 2025, https://www.youtube.com/watch?v=-SD_MucCa6c
6. Rosemary M. Wixom "As individuals we are strong. Together, with God, we are unstoppable.", accessed August 28,2025, https://www.churchofjesuschrist.org/media/image/meme-wixom-together-482cb70?lang=eng
7. Oxford Reference, 'self-care' reworded, accessed August 28, 2025, https://www.oxfordreference.com/display/10.1093/oi/authority.20110803100453172
8. Bible Hub, 'Soul-Care' reworded, accessed August 28, 2025, https://biblehub.com/q/what_is_soul_care.htm

9. Manchester Metropolitan University, accessed September 20, 2025, https://www.mmu.ac.uk/
10. PRINCE2, accessed September 20, 2025 https://www.prince2.com/uk/prince2?gad_source=1&gad_campaignid=22310643829&gbraid=0AAAAAD_o0S0PRrUlhy3EFEp4I0uNr9b9t&gclid=CjwKCAjwobnGBhBNEiwAu2mpFPOvXFrQAi2vDQgo43HsP9vVPbKBOgCr_iwv-osYX3fGyv1IhPahehoCBcQQAvD_BwE
11. YouVersion, accessed September 20, 2025, https://www.youversion.com/
12. HOW TO START 2024 SUCCESSFULLY: 2024 goal setting template, vision, reinvent yourself, & mindset!, accessed September 20, 2025, https://www.youtube.com/watch?v=RUOB33AYVgU
13. Legal Imposters, accessed September 20, 2025, https://www.amazon.co.uk/Legal-Imposters/dp/B0BNBTJ84W?dplnkId=7cde6935-33ff-4af1-a797-66cb1ad54103
14. Don't Drop the Call X Sarah Jakes Roberts, accessed September 20, 2025 https://youtu.be/e__nXbwUaNE?si=nHBbYZBlvfu1B__o
15. Fitness Holiday, accessed September 20, 2025, https://www.fitnwild.com/events-holidays
16. Five Stages of Business Growth, accessed September 20, 2025, https://generic.wordpress.soton.ac.uk/meetingofminds/2018/05/03/five-stages-of-business-growth/
17. Hillsong Church, accessed September 20, 2025, https://hillsong.com/uk/

18. Vinted, accessed September 20, 2025, https://www.vinted.co.uk/
19. Romans 12:12,ESV, accessed September 19, 2025, https://www.biblestudytools.com/romans/12-12.html
20. James 1:2-4,NIV, accessed September 19, 2025, https://www.biblestudytools.com/james/passage/?q=james+1:2-4
21. Colossians 3:23,NIV, accessed September 19, 2025, https://www.biblestudytools.com/colossians/3-23.html
22. Isaiah 41:10,NIV, accessed September 19, 2025, https://www.biblestudytools.com/isaiah/41-10.html
23. Ephesians 4:29,NIV, accessed September 19, 2025, https://www.biblestudytools.com/ephesians/4-29.html
24. Hebrews 10:24-25,NIV, accessed September 20, 2025, https://www.biblestudytools.com/hebrews/passage/?q=hebrews+10:24-25
25. Proverbs 16:9,ESV, accessed September 20, 2025, https://www.biblestudytools.com/esv/proverbs/16-9.html
26. Proverbs 15:22,ESV, accessed September 20, 2025, https://www.biblestudytools.com/esv/proverbs/15-22.html
27. Proverbs 19:21,ESV, accessed September 20, 2025, https://www.biblestudytools.com/esv/proverbs/19-21.html
28. 2 Timothy 1:7,NIV, accessed September 20, 2025, https://www.biblestudytools.com/2-timothy/1-7.html

29. Proverbs 16:3,NIV, accessed September 20, 2025, https://www.biblestudytools.com/proverbs/16-3.html
30. Deuteronomy 31:6,ESV, accessed September 20, 2025, https://www.biblestudytools.com/esv/deuteronomy/31-6.html
31. Romans 15:13,NIV, accessed September 20, 2025, https://www.biblestudytools.com/romans/15-13.html
32. Jeremiah 29:11,NIV, accessed September 20, 2025, https://www.biblestudytools.com/jeremiah/29-11.html
33. 1 Peter 5:7,NIV, accessed September 20, 2025, https://www.biblestudytools.com/1-peter/5-7.html
34. Corinthians 3:16,ESV, accessed September 20, 2025, https://www.biblestudytools.com/esv/1-corinthians/3-16.html
35. Psalms 46:5,NIV, accessed September 20, 2025, https://www.biblestudytools.com/psalms/46-5.html
36. Philippians 4:6-8,ESV, accessed September 20, 2025, https://www.biblestudytools.com/esv/philippians/4.html
37. 1 Timothy 6:10,NIV, accessed September 20, 2025, https://www.biblestudytools.com/1-timothy/6-10.html
38. 2 Corinthians 9:6,NIV, accessed September 20, 2025, https://www.biblestudytools.com/2-corinthians/9-6.html
39. Deuteronomy 8:18,NIV, accessed September 20, 2025, https://www.biblestudytools.com/deuteronomy/8-18.html

40. Matthew 6:33,ESV, accessed September 20, 2025, https://www.biblestudytools.com/esv/matthew/6-33.html
41. 2 Corinthians 6:11-13,NIV, accessed September 20, 2025, https://www.biblestudytools.com/2-corinthians/passage/?q=2+corinthians+6:11-13
42. Matthew 21:22,NIV, accessed September 20, 2025, https://www.biblestudytools.com/matthew/21-22.html
43. Genesis 2:18,NIV, accessed September 20, 2025, https://www.biblestudytools.com/genesis/2-18.html
44. Proverbs 27:17,NIV, accessed September 20, 2025, https://www.biblestudytools.com/proverbs/27-17.html
45. Acts 7:38,NIV, accessed September 20, 2025, https://www.biblestudytools.com/acts/7-38.html
46. Psalms 139:14,NIV, accessed September 20, 2025, https://www.biblestudytools.com/psalms/139-14.html
47. Ecclesiastes 3:1-8,NIV, accessed September 20, 2025, https://www.biblestudytools.com/ecclesiastes/passage/?q=ecclesiastes+3:1-8
48. 1 Corinthians 13:4-8,NIV, accessed September 20, 2025, https://www.biblestudytools.com/1-corinthians/passage/?q=1+corinthians+13:4-8
49. 1 Corinthians 6:19-20,NIV, accessed September 20, 2025, https://www.biblestudytools.com/1-corinthians/passage/?q=1+corinthians+6:19-20
50. Matthew 11:28,NIV, accessed September 20, 2025, https://www.biblestudytools.com/matthew/11-28.html

51. Proverbs 4:23,NIV, accessed September 20, 2025, https://www.biblestudytools.com/proverbs/4-23.html
52. Luke 8:15,NIV, accessed September 20, 2025, https://www.biblestudytools.com/luke/8-15.html
53. Wikipedia, 'self-discipline' accessed November 2, 2025, https://en.wikipedia.org/wiki/Discipline
54. Cambridge Dictionary, 'consistency', accessed November 2, 2025, https://dictionary.cambridge.org/dictionary/english/consistency
55. Bazaar, 10 simple steps to being more sustainable, accessed November 2, 2025, https://www.harpersbazaar.com/uk/fashion/shopping/a41158/how-to-be-sustainable-fashion/
56. Bible Hub, Learning in the Wilderness, accessed November 2, 2025, https://biblehub.com/topical/l/learning_in_the_wilderness.htm#:~:text=The%20Israelites%20learned%20dependence%20on%20God%20for,a%20period%20of%20learning%20in%20the%20wilderness
57. Montelle Bee, PLAN My 12-Week Year With Me! *Updated Notion Template* Q2 Goal Planning + Reset, accessed November 2, 2025, https://youtu.be/2t4bijkDyLI?si=rHERyIqatL9PyZTP)
58. Caroline Flanagan, Episode 2 - What Exactly is Imposter Syndrome (10 November 2022), Legal Imposters, accessed November 2, 2025, https://www.amazon.co.uk/Legal-Imposters/dp/B0BNBTJ84W?dplnkId=7cde6935-33ff-4af1-a797-66cb1ad54103

www.ingramcontent.com/pod-product-compliance
Lightning Source LLC
LaVergne TN
LVHW011203080426
835508LV00007B/571